The LDS Gospel of
LIGHT

By

B. Grant Bishop, M.D.

First published by Ponce de Leon
telephone: 1–801–298–9890

Copyright © B. Grant Bishop, 1998

All rights reserved

ISBN 0–9668360–1–4

Printed in the United States of America

PUBLISHER'S NOTE
Without limiting the rights under copyright reserved above, no part of this publication may be reproduced, stored in or introduced into a retrieval system, or transmitted in any form or by any means (electronic, mechanical, photocopying, recording, or otherwise), without the prior written permission of both the copyright owner and the above publisher of this book.

Acknowledgments

I cannot remember a time when I did not know and believe the Joseph Smith story, or a moment when I doubted the truthfulness of the restored gospel of Jesus Christ. My good parents taught me the gospel of Jesus Christ through songs, stories, and example. They planted in me the desire to search for truth, and from them I learned the excitement that comes from discovering my environment through heart and mind. To them I am most grateful.

I have had wonderful opportunities to share the gospel of Jesus Christ through word and spirit. I am grateful to those who have given me the challenge of teaching. There is a contagious spirit in seeing the excitement in others when they learn and feel the spirit of truth.

Mark Taylor and Keith Terry gave me the challenge and the opportunity to put my thoughts into a book, and my friend Arvin Gibson helped me through the process. Thank you.

Dedicated to

Nelda,

who has always lived the gospel of Jesus Christ
through her heart.

Contents

GOD THE FATHER

1. The Glory of God 1
2. God and the Nature of Light 9
3. The Mystery of God, Light, and Matter 23
4. God and His Attributes 31
5. Near-Death Experiences and God's Light 45

JESUS CHRIST
HOLY GHOST

6. Jesus Christ: Expression of the Father 55
7. Holy Ghost: Dispenser of Light 67

8. Creation: the Ordering of Light 75

9. Jesus Christ: God of Light Comes to Earth 89

CHILDREN OF LIGHT

10. Children of Light/Children of Darkness 105

11. Children of Light: Facing Darkness 119

12. Children of Light: Coming to the Light of Christ . 135

13. Children of Light: Becoming the Light of Christ . 151

14. Children of Light: Becoming Gods of Light 165

15. Wholeness 177

REFERENCES

Appendices 189

References 213

Index 235

Part I

GOD THE FATHER

Chapter 1
The Glory of God

"God is light" (1 John 1:5)

GOD'S GLORY

Our Father is not just a being *with* light. He *is* light itself. God is light! He is light in all its glory and majesty. It is not a metaphor any more than "Christ is the Savior of the world" is a metaphor. It is his light which is his love, and it is his light which encompasses all his being, power, and attributes, and it is therefore light which we should study and experience to more fully understand our Father. Any study of physical light would be incomplete without including a study of God's light. God and light are as inseparable as Christ and salvation. Comprehending light is comprehending God.

What we receive from God is light because "that which is of God is light; and he that receiveth light, and continueth in God, receiveth more light; and that light groweth brighter and brighter until the perfect day."[1] However, only a small fraction of the light we receive is visual. Most light is non-visual. Besides perceiving light with our eyes, we receive light with our minds, with our spirits, and with our hearts, and yet all are variations of the light of God. All truth, including love, is light from God. Truth comes to us from God through many forms of physical and spiritual light.

Those who have seen God have always described their experience in terms of light and glory, glory and light being synonymous terms. "The *glory* of God is intelligence or, in other words, *light* and *truth*."[2] From Paul, who saw "a great light round about,"[3] to Steven, who "saw the glory of God,"[4] to Joseph Smith, who "saw a pillar of light . . . [containing] two Personages, whose brightness and glory defy all description,"[5] all have had as the centerpiece of their experience the glory and light of God. Joseph Smith, along with Oliver Cowdery, saw God and declared, "his countenance shone above the brightness of the sun."[6] In January 1836 Joseph Smith and others saw "the celestial kingdom of God and the glory thereof. . . . the transcendent beauty of the gate . . . like unto circling flames of fire; also the blazing throne of God, whereon was seated the Father and the Son."[7]

In Moses's inspiring experience with our Father's light, the power of God lifted him to a mountain top where God's glory came upon him and he saw the face of God. God told him that "no man can behold all my works, except he behold all my glory; and no man can behold all my glory, and afterwards remain in the flesh . . . for my works are without end . . . and I will show thee the workmanship of mine hands; but not all."[8] Since God's glory is his works which cannot be totally comprehended in the flesh, part of his glorious light is beyond our capacity to see or feel. It is larger than human understanding. With God's glorious light upon him, Moses beheld not only the creation of the world, but the end of the world as well, and all the history of the children of men.

After God withdrew from Moses, "Satan came tempting," and Moses declared to Satan that he, Moses, was "a son of God, in the similitude of his Only Begotten." Moses then made this important comparison between Satan and God: "Where is thy glory" Moses asked Satan, "that I should worship thee . . . for it is *darkness* unto me?"[9] Moses could not look upon God except God's glory came upon him and transfigured him, but he could look upon Satan as a natural man. Moses told Satan he could judge between "thee and God: for God said unto me: Worship God, for him only shalt thou serve. Get thee hence, Satan; deceive me not; for God said unto me: Thou art after the similitude of mine Only Begotten."[10]

After Satan disappeared, the glory of God rested upon Moses again and he beheld the earth, "even all of it; and there was not a particle of it which he did not behold, *discerning it by the spirit of God.*" Moses beheld also the innumerable inhabitants of the earth "and there was not a soul which he beheld not." The Lord God then spake unto Moses, saying, "The heavens, they are many, and they cannot be numbered unto man, but they are numbered unto me, for they are mine. And as one earth shall pass away, and the heavens thereof even so shall another come: and there is no end to my works, neither to my words. For behold, *this is my work and my glory*—to bring to pass the immortality and eternal life of man."[11]

By judging the difference between God's glory and Satan's darkness, Moses understood his true nature and his relationship with God. It was by the light of God's glory that Moses saw the creation of the earth, all its particles, its end and its inhabitants. God's glory is his creations, which will go on forever. We are the most important part of God's work. We are sons and daughters, in similitude of God's Only Begotten.

EVERLASTING BURNINGS

After revealing the refining power of God's light, Isaiah asked, "Who among us shall dwell with the devouring fire? who among us shall dwell with everlasting burnings?"[12] This devouring fire is a theme repeated often and describes not only God's destructive power, but also the purifying power of God's light, which will cleanse us from all darkness. Joseph Smith prayed that Christ should "rend the heavens . . . and come down, that the mountains might flow down at [his] presence." When Christ answers and comes, he "shall be as the melting fire that burneth, and as the fire which causeth the waters to boil." All nations will tremble at Christ's presence, and "so great shall be the glory of his presence that the sun shall hide his face in shame, and the moon shall withhold its light, and the stars shall be hurled from their places."[13]

Joseph Smith taught, "God Almighty Himself dwells in eternal fire; flesh and blood cannot go there, for all corruption is devoured by the fire. Our God is a consuming fire. . . . Immortality dwells in everlasting burnings. . . . All men who are immortal dwell in everlasting burnings."[14] What power will come upon us! Before we come into the presence of God, our imperfections will have been consumed by the purifying fire of God, leaving only the holy and pure within us.

God's light is perfect and will not tolerate darkness and therefore God's cleansing power must remove all darkness in us before we can come into his presence. "And Moses went up into the mount. . . . And the glory of the Lord abode upon mount Sinai, . . . And the sight of the glory of the Lord was like devouring fire on the top of the mount."[15] Moses explained, "But now mine own eyes have beheld God; but not my natural, but my spiritual eyes, for my natural eyes could not have beheld; for I should have withered and died in his presence; but his glory was upon me; and I beheld his face, for I was transfigured before him."[16]

Joseph Smith ends his overpowering revelation of the Celestial Kingdom by declaring how "great and marvelous are the works of the Lord, and the mysteries of his kingdom." The Celestial Kingdom surpasses "all understanding in glory, and in might, and in dominion," and it can only be understood "by the power of the Holy Spirit, which God bestows on those who love him. . . . To whom he grants this privilege of seeing and knowing for themselves; That through the power and manifestation of the Spirit, while in the flesh, they may be able to bear his presence in the world of glory. And to God and the Lamb be glory, and honor, and dominion forever and ever. Amen."[17] If not while we are in the flesh, then surely in the resurrected body, God's purifying fire will cleanse us of our imperfections, permitting us to comprehend his light and his glory, "for our God is a consuming fire."[18]

WE CAN RECEIVE GOD'S GLORY

The overwhelming insight which Moses received from God was an understanding of the purpose of life. Moses learned that God wants to share his light and glory with us, immortalize us, and guide us to celestial life.[19] Like Moses, we are also sons and daughters of God, in similitude of his Only Begotten. We also were "in the beginning with God." We are "intelligence, or the light of truth, [and we were] not created or made, neither indeed can be."[20] This is such an important revelation. We are part of God's glory and have always been with him. The beautiful truth of the gospel of light is that we are the intimate part of his work. God wants to dress us in layers of light, so we may partake in the whole of his glory! This is our Father's great gift which he yearns to share with each of us.

Christ told Joseph Smith to prepare for the gathering and the building of Zion, that " all things shall become new and my knowledge and glory may dwell upon all the earth . . . that the wheat may be secured in the garners to posses eternal life, and be crowned with celestial glory."[21] We, like Moses, are promised celestial glory when we come into God's light. "And to them will I reveal all mysteries, yea all the hidden mysteries of my kingdom from days of old, and for ages to come, will I make known unto them the good pleasure of my will concerning all things pertaining to my kingdom. Yea, even the wonders of eternity shall they know, and things to come will I show them, even the things of many generations."[22] The revelation of all things is the "glory of the celestial," which glory Joseph Smith and Sidney Rigdon saw in January of 1832. "And thus we saw . . . where God, even the Father, reigns upon his throne forever and ever."[23] Celestial glory is the promise of Jesus Christ, the Second Comforter. "This Comforter is the promise which I give unto you of eternal life, even the glory of the celestial kingdom."[24] Celestial glory is rest, which is the fullness of his glory.[25] The restored gospel makes it clear that our goal should be nothing short of celestial glory, promised us by God. Celestial glory is making the light of Jesus Christ live within us.

VARIATIONS OF GOD'S LIGHT

Tied into the glory of God are all the expressions of love that come from him, including life itself, for God is "the light which shineth which giveth [us] *light.*"[26] "[For] in Him was life; and the *life* was the light of men."[27] Light is the essence of our very beings, our *intelligence*.[28] Light is the *law* by which all things are governed,[29] and the *judgment* by which we live.[30] Light is *truth*, *spirit*, and the *word*. Light is the *spirit of Christ* that cares for our spirits as our *consciences*. "For the *word* of the Lord is *truth*, and whatsoever is *truth is light*, and whatsoever is *light is Spirit*, even *the Spirit of Jesus Christ*. And the Spirit giveth light to every man that cometh into the world."[31] Light is *knowledge, understanding,* and *the everlasting gospel*.[32] "Light . . . is in all things, . . . even *the power of God* who sitteth upon his throne."[33] That power includes *priesthood* which the sons of Aaron and Moses received as glory,[34] and it includes all the soft attributes of the spirit of God such as *mercy, virtue,* and *compassion*.[35]

There are many manifestations of spiritual light, the Glory of God, expressed to us through different flavors, feelings and inspiration. Light is visual and non-visual, physical and spiritual, powerful and creative, peaceful and healing, loving and eternal. Light has been within us forever because our intelligences are light. Light will be with us through eternity because celestial glory is light. Light is in our beings, our spirits and the life of our bodies. Light is the glory of God. Light is the love of God. Light is God!

Chapter 2
God and the Nature of Light

"He is in the sun, and the light of the sun" (D&C 88:7)
"There is no such thing as immaterial matter" (D&C 131:7)

The new scientific discoveries about our universe, about light, time and space can give meaning to what the scriptures reveal about God, the author of light. Scientific knowledge about light clarifies what the scriptures say about us, the creation, and the veil. In 1613, coming under judgment from the Inquisition, Galileo wrote to his friend Father Castelli, "The task of wise interpreters is to find meaning in scriptural passages that will agree with the evidence of sensory experience. . . . Holy scripture and nature proceed equally from the Divine Word, the former by the Holy Spirit, the latter as a very faithful execution of God's order."[1]

Our scientific knowledge is always changing, renewing itself with new-found information, sometimes clarifying old ideas and sometimes revealing facts never before thought of.

Most of what I learned as a medical student 30 years ago is completely outdated. Never has there been a time with so many scientific discoveries and such exciting visions of our universe. Both our spiritual world and physical world come from a loving Father. Current scientific knowledge can bring new meaning to scripture, making the word of God and the actual physical creations of God more compatible. Likewise our spiritual experiences can increase our understanding about our physical world.

As we will see, light has two forms, with each form having different characteristics. Since we live in a universe made up of light, understanding the dual nature of light can help us understand our universe. Since God is light,[2] God should exhibit both forms of light and have the characteristics of each form. The gospel of Jesus Christ is a gospel of light. Therefore, it should express both forms of light. Since we are the children of God, our nature should also be like God's, having both forms of light. We are spirit and body, heart and mind. Part of resolving the puzzle of life centers on uniting the two different parts of our being into one whole. It is clear that God the Father and Jesus Christ are beings of light, and therefore their gospel of light should show us how the two forms of light unite into one whole.

Just as no mortal really understands the light and power of God, no scientist fully understands the nature of light. But the scientific characteristics of physical light can be compared to what the scriptures, near-death experiences and heavenly visions teach us about the light, power and glory of God. A study of light is not just the study of what we see with our eyes, nor is it limited to the study of what we know scientifically. A study of light includes a study of energy, matter, creation, intelligence, life, love, grace, compassion, knowledge, priesthood, celestial kingdoms, death, sorrow, judgment, laws, opposites, and resurrection. How the atonement works and how we take advantage of it is a subject of light. The gospel of light can teach us about the positive and loving aspects of the judgment, and it can give us understanding of how light can literally fill every tiny space in our being, potentially cleansing and lifting us back into the bosom of our Heavenly Father.

THE ELECTROMAGNETIC SPECTRUM

God's power is his glory and light. His power makes things happen, whether by creating a universe, overcoming evil, or holding us with mercy and love. God's power will produce some change either in matter, spirit or intelligence. When God said, "Let there be light," he released upon the void his personal power of light, and through his light everything was created. Joseph Smith was told that Christ is the light in the sun and stars, as well as the power by which they were made.[3] Joseph was also taught that Christ is *"the light which is in all things*, which [gives] *life* to all things, which is the *law* by which all things are governed, even the *power of God.*"[4] These scriptures reveal that light, life, and law are synonymous with the power of God.

In science, light is a form of energy. Light, energy, mass, force, work, and power are all interrelated. *Energy* is the ability to do work, and *work* is the *force* exerted on an object times the distance the object moves. *Power* is measured by how fast the work is accomplished. There are only four known forces in the universe—gravity, strong nuclear force, weak nuclear force, and electromagnetic force. *Gravity* is the force that matter has which attracts other matter. It keeps us bound to earth and governs how planets, satellites and stars move in the heavens. It is gravity which governs the vast spaces of the universe. It is the force which compresses gases into nebulae which then become galaxies and solar systems.

The other three forces are related to each other and are thought to be variations of a single force. They create orderliness in the atom, allowing elements and compounds to form as building blocks for matter and life. The *strong nuclear force* holds neutrons and protons in the nucleus so the atom doesn't fly apart. Huge amounts of energy can be produced by separating, or joining nuclear components to form energy, just as Einstein's equation predicts. It is the energy of atomic and hydrogen bombs, and the energy which powers the stars. The *weak nuclear force* helps bind the electron in the atom and causes some parts of the atom to break away spontaneously.

The *electromagnetic force* holds the electrons circling around the nucleus in their orbits. Whenever an electron changes its orbit around an atom to one nearer the nucleus, energy is released and a photon of light is emitted, which can be observed as visible light. Atoms connect with each other by sharing their electrons, producing orderly interaction to form groups of molecules and compounds, and allowing matter to act in a predictable manner. Visual light is only a small portion of electromagnetic energy.[5]

All electromagnetic energy acts like waves, similar to the waves in the ocean, or the waves that are produced if you drop a rock into a pond of water. Waves have crests and troughs, and they come in variable lengths. The length of a wave is measured from the top of one crest to the top of the next crest. The distance between two ocean waves could be several meters, or as small as a few centimeters. Some electromagnetic energy waves are so small we have to measure them in nanometers (nm).[6]

In the range of visual electromagnetic light energy, the only difference between colors of light is the length of their waves. Likewise, the only difference between visual and nonvisual light is the length of their waves. Just outside of the visual spectrum of light there is infrared light with longer waves, and ultraviolet light with shorter waves. But the electromagnetic spectrum is continuous. It includes gamma and x-rays on the short side, and radio, short wave radio and microwaves on the long side. The only thing that is different about them is their wave lengths, which also determines the amount of energy each produces.

The electromagnetic spectrum can be compared to the spectrum of sound. All notes are sound waves. The only difference between different sounds is the length of their waves. Some sound waves are so long or so short that we do not hear them. We label different sounds with different names according to their pitch, such as a "C" note or a "G" note. All the energy along the electromagnetic spectrum is made up of the same thing. We just label one wave length a radio wave or a gamma wave because they have different effects, just as a "C" note has a different pitch than a "G" note. We are receiving a variation of the same thing whether we are getting a sunburn, having a broken arm x-rayed, or seeing a beautiful sunset. The different results that occur from the varied waves come because each varied wave has a different energy level associated with it. The shorter the wave, the higher the energy. Since visual light just happens to be one variation of electromagnetic energy, "light" in this work is used not only as a general term describing all energy along the electromagnetic spectrum, but it is also used as a general term to designate the power, glory, love, and light of God.

Light energy warms and cooks our food in microwaves. It burns our skin as ultraviolet waves. It helps us communicate through radios, fiber optics, and laser operated satellites. It is the source of electricity and the source of all chemical reactions including the production of oxygen from plants. Light energy controls the price scanners in our stores, and plays our CDs and operates our security systems. As lasers it is used for the healing of our bodies and in weapon systems for the destruction of our bodies. Both ends of the electromagnetic spectrum are open. Scientists expect that there will be new forms of energy discovered in the future which will be part of the electromagnetic spectrum.

Just as electromagnetic energy includes both visual and nonvisual light which produce different reactions with matter and spirit, the light of God includes a whole spectrum of power, both seen and unseen, which also causes different reactions with matter and spirit. Joseph Smith was told that Christ is, " in all things, the light of truth."[7] To make sure Joseph didn't misunderstand and conclude that Christ's light is only spiritual, Joseph was told that Christ is in the sun, the moon and the stars. Christ was the light of the sun, moon and stars and the power by which they were made; "And the earth also, and the power thereof, even the earth upon which you stand. *And the light which shineth, which giveth you light, is through him who enlighteneth your eyes, which is the same light that quickeneth your understandings.*"[8]

The light which shines into our eyes is the same light that gives our souls understanding! Heart-warming spiritual light therefore must also be a form of energy. The energy of the electromagnetic spectrum apparently is but a small part of the spectrum of God's light. The light of God and Christ — life, intelligence, immortality, laws, truth, spirit, words, conscience, knowledge, understanding, the everlasting gospel, mercy, virtue, compassion, rest, and peace may, indeed, just be different lengths of the same energy scientists have named gamma rays, x-rays, ultraviolet light, visual light, infrared light, short wave radio waves, radio waves and microwaves. That means the warmth that comes from the light of the sun is just a variation of the warmth that comes from holding a loved one. The energy produced by an electric power plant is only a variation of the energy given and received in a priesthood blessing. The lighting of a beautiful city is but a visual expression of the compassionate light felt by a sorrowing loved one. All the medical knowledge which helps heal the sick is but a simple form of the atoning power of Christ that heals not only bodies but our souls.

Perhaps the only difference between the different types of *spiritual light* is their wave lengths. There is energy that is radiated into our skin when ultraviolet light burns us, and there is real energy that is radiated into our hearts when we are touched by the light of Christ. Perhaps the open ends of the electromagnetic spectrum are occupied by the varied expressions of the light of God and all of it comes under the energy and power of God called glory, love and light.

The force of electromagnetism, which includes the strong and weak forces of the nucleus, is the light power of the universe, and it seems reasonable that it also encompasses the physical expressions of the power of God. The physical forces of the universe govern its laws, bringing reliability in the performance of the basic elements. The speed of light is consistent throughout the cosmos. Just like the laws of God, the laws that regulate time and space don't vary. Are the laws of physics part of the light of God *"which is the law by which all things are governed, even the power of God who sitteth upon his throne, who is in the bosom of eternity?"*[9] Christ told Joseph Smith that there is no part of the universe which does not abide law, nor any space in the universe where there is no matter or energy.[10]

Since the energy of physical light depends on its wave length, we need different instruments to detect different types of energy. A radio won't pick up an x-ray of our chest, nor do we plug in a hair blower to make a telephone call. Gamma rays will not operate a short wave radio, but will do a very fine job in creating cancer. There are million dollar telescopes, some miles in width, trying to detect different aspects of the universe, from subatomic particles to supernovas. We cannot comprehend our universe with just one instrument. Likewise, we cannot comprehend the full measure of the light of God using just one aspect of our being. Our senses are instruments that detect different presentations of our universe. We learn the letter of the law with our minds, and the spirit of the law with our souls. Understanding the logic of justice will not always help us feel mercy and compassion. Just as studying the physical universe requires our creative power to discover all that exists, studying the gospel of light requires all our powers to detect and feel the fullness of its reality.

DICHOTOMY OF LIGHT

We know that light has the characteristics of waves because light produces a phenomenon called interference. Interference patterns occur when two or more waves run into each other and *interfere* with the initial waves. To illustrate, if two stones were dropped a few feet apart in a still pool of water, each stone would produce rings of waves. Where the waves run into each other, an interference pattern develops. Where the crests of two waves hit, the effect is a larger wave, and where a crest and a trough hit, they cancel each other. This interaction of waves forms a complex arrangement of alternating crests and troughs. With light waves, the interference pattern is seen as alternating bands of light and dark in a complex pattern.[11] Everything in the universe emits vibrating waves, not only light and all subatomic particles, but also cars, bowling balls, rocks, and humans.

However, light does not express itself only in a wave form. Light also comes in a second form, a particle form. But waves and particles have different properties. While waves are weightless, infinite, continuous, and spread out, particles have weight (mass) and are small, finite, discrete, and individual. The particle form of light does not produce an interference pattern but a photoelectric pattern. In the particle form, light acts like tiny individual bullets, which, if shot at a plate of film, leave discrete, isolated white spots.[12] Light thus has a dual nature. It is a dichotomy, acting as both wave and particle. This dual nature occurs not only with visual light but with all forms of light on the electromagnetic spectrum, including gamma rays, X rays, and radio waves.

The wave/particle dichotomy is also characteristic of all subatomic matter. For example, if an electron, acting like a particle, is shot at a piece of glass coated with phosphorescent chemicals, the electron will leave a small point of light. Our televisions work by shooting thousands of electrons at such a piece of glass. But electrons and all other subatomic particles can also dissolve into a cloud of energy and behave as if they were waves spread throughout the universe. What is even stranger is that they are not just a wave at one time and a particle at another time, but are really both at the same time. It would be like seeing smooth waves of water hit a sandy beach, change instantaneously to individual droplets of water, pulsating onto the shore, and then change back again into waves before we know it.

When viewed from a subatomic level, all matter is just a variation of light, having similar dichotomous forms of wave and particle, and therefore, everything in the universe is ultimately related to light. Melvin Morse, M.D., from his book *Transformed by the Light*, says that until fifty years ago, scientists thought atoms were composed only of electrons, protons and neutrons:

> Then science discovered an even smaller world than the electron. They call this tiny world wave/particle duality.

According to astrophysicist Stephen Hawking, it works like this: As physicists have split the atom into smaller and smaller particles, they have discovered to their surprise that there is no final 'tiniest part' of nature. Rather, *there are forces best described as wavelengths of electromagnetism, or light. These pieces of light serve as the fundamental building blocks for everything. What this theory tells us is that everything we consider to be real actually breaks down into simple light, in all of its various wavelengths.*[13]

LIGHT IS ETERNAL MATTER

Light, energy and mass (how much an object weighs) are related as expressed in Einstein's famous equation $E=mc^2$. Energy equals the mass of physical matter times the speed of light squared. In other words, energy and matter are two forms of the same thing! That is important. Light is energy and energy can be changed into matter. That means everything in the universe is a variation of light.

God said, "The elements are eternal,"[14] and Joseph Smith taught, "Anything created cannot be eternal; and earth, water, etc., had their existence in an elementary state, from eternity."[15] Joseph also taught, "Elements had an existence from the time [God] had. . . . [Elements] can never be destroyed; they may be organized and re-organized but not destroyed. They had no beginning and can have no end."[16] Parley P. Pratt stated, there is "a boundless infinitude of space," where there "exists all the varieties of the elements, properties, or things of which intelligence takes cognizance," and where "the elements of all these properties or things are eternal, uncreated, self-existing. Not one particle can be added to them by creative power; neither can one particle be diminished or annihilated."[17] Amazingly, Joseph Smith and Parley P. Pratt, some sixty years before Einstein discovered relativity, taught that matter cannot be destroyed. Matter can only change its form into energy and then back to matter again. There is no loss of matter or energy in the universe. There is a constant total of "stuff" in the universe which can only change its form from energy to matter and back again.

Not only is light energy and energy a form of matter, but our uncreated intelligences are light.[18] Our spirits are matter, but our spirits are "more pure, elastic and refined matter than the body."[19] Since our spirits are matter they also are a form of light. God said, that "whatsoever is truth is light, and whatsoever is light is Spirit, even the Spirit of Jesus Christ."[20] Our intelligences are dressed with more light called spiritual matter, and then dressed again with the light of eternal matter to form our physical bodies.

In gospel terms, intelligence, spirit, matter, elements, and law are described as separate entities because they have different properties, but they are all variations of light. They are all variations of God's light and love. In scientific terms, visual light, X-ray, radio waves, and sub-atomic particles are described as separate entities because they have different properties, but they are all variations of light. They all obey God's law in their own kingdom,[21] whether spiritual or physical, whether acting as wave or particle, energy or matter. What we call the laws of physics are probably just a portion of the physical laws of God. Just as we don't understand fully what physical light is, we also only have an elementary understanding of the light of God. Even though we only have a Kindergarten knowledge as to how physical law fits into

God's kingdom, the similarities between energy/matter, wave/particle and spirit/matter can help us understand the reality of our spirit and physical worlds.

Chapter 3
The Mystery of God, Light, and Matter

"The brother of Jared . . . saw the finger of the Lord"
(Ether 3:6)

THE STRANGENESS OF LIGHT AND MATTER

The reality of our universe is that truth has two opposite forms. Light and subatomic parts are both wave and particle. Light is energy. Matter is also energy, so matter is just light in another form. In the first part of this century when the nature of light and matter was being discovered, it was not easy for scientists to believe that both light and subatomic parts are both wave and particle. It would have been easier to accept one form of reality and not two contradictory forms. But two forms of light and matter are what scientists found and that is what they had to accept. It took years of research for scientists to finally accept the fact that both forms of reality were scientifically provable. Truth is two things and not one, and the reason for the differences still cannot be explained.

There is even more strangeness to the story of light and matter, a strangeness still not understood by scientists. But it is a strangeness that will sound very familiar to those who believe that God gives life to everything and that God's light is throughout the expanse of space.

From a scientific point, matter seems to have life, not only because there is a wave/particle duality to nature but also because subatomic parts have an amazing ability to be interconnected, to communicate with each other, and to act as a unified whole. Because of the way electrons are interconnected they appear to be communicating faster than the speed of light, as if there were no time or space separating them. It is possible for one electron to communicate with a second electron instantly even when they are miles apart. Under certain conditions, a high density of electrons act like one whole, similar to a flock of birds changing directions in flight all at the same time.[1]

One physicist, David Bohm, was so impressed with how electrons act that he remarked that they actually seemed to be *alive*.[2] Bohm said that "dividing the universe up into living and nonliving things . . . has no meaning. Animate and inanimate matter are inseparably interwoven, and life, too, . . . [is spread] throughout the totality of the universe. Even a rock is in some way alive . . . for life and intelligence are present not only in all of matter, but in 'energy,' 'space,' time,' 'the fabric of the entire universe.'"[3]

Modern physics supports the concept that there is *life* in all matter and that the entire universe is connected in some way.[4] Fred Hoyle, one of the important pioneers in modern astronomy, wrote, "Present day development in cosmology are coming to suggest rather insistently that everyday conditions could not persist but for the distant parts of the Universe, that all our ideas of space and geometry would become entirely invalid if the distant parts of the Universe were taken away. Our everyday experience even down to the smallest details seems to be so closely integrated to the grand-scale features of the Universe that it is well-nigh impossible to contemplate the two being separate."[5] The modern physics of light and matter reveal that we are connected in someway with the entire universe. In summarizing the new physics, Gary Zukav wrote, "The philosophical implication of quantum mechanics is that all of the things in our universe (including us) that appear to exist independently are actually parts of one all-encompassing organic pattern, and that no parts of the pattern are ever really separate from it or from each other."[6]

Could there be anything stranger than that there is life in all matter and that the entire universe is connected? As strange as that sounds, it is not only supported by scientists, but by modern prophets who taught those ideas some fifty years before quantum physics was even known. Brigham Young taught, "There is not a particle of element which is not filled with life, and all space is filled with element; there is no such thing as empty space. . . . Life in various proportions, combinations, conditions &c., fills all matter. . . . There is life in all matter, throughout the vast extent of all the eternities; it is in the rock, the sand, the dust, in water, air, the gases, and, in short, in every description and organization of matter, whether it be solid, liquid, or gaseous."[7] Brigham Young also suggested that the entire universe is connected through the divine nature of God. "Eternity is without bounds, and is filled with matter; and there is no such place as empty space. . . . There is an eternity of matter, and it is all acted upon and filled with a portion of divinity . . . organized . . . into animals, vegetables, and into intelligent beings."[8]

This universal light of life which is in everything would include the earth as explained by Orson Pratt. "I think if one could see a little further, we would understand that, connected with the materials of the earth is a living principle, a principle too, that acts according to certain laws, intelligently, not blindly; and that our earth, in performing its course, following the track marked out, does so according to law."[9] Christ told Joseph Smith, "[T]he earth abideth the law of a celestial kingdom, for it filleth the measure of its creation, and transgresseth not the law." And as a living body, the earth "shall die, [and] it shall be quickened again, and shall abide the power by which it is quickened, and the righteous shall inherit it."[10]

SPIRIT AND MATTER

In the physical world which we are most used to, matter behaves as though it is restricted to a given place and a given time. That is the world in which Isaac Newton's laws of physics predict the behavior of nature, and the only world which was thought to exist prior to the twentieth century. But in the subatomic world of quantum mechanics, light, matter and energy are not so restricted. Our universe is continually expressing itself as wave and particle, energy and matter. For example, our bodies seem to be solid but in reality we are organized energy, vibrating between wave and matter. Our bodies are in a flux, recreating ourselves every second, powered by light, spirit and intelligence, having 6 trillion reactions occur every second in each of our 70 trillion cells. Our atoms, including oxygen, carbon and hydrogen, are being broken down and reorganized constantly and then rearranged into other compounds, rejuvenating all parts of our bodies. Our skin turns over every forty days. Our skeletons are rebuilt in three months. Our livers take six weeks to renew themselves. We look solid just as the moving propellers of an airplane look solid. Our atoms are moving so fast we only seem solid, but in our case even the atoms are renewing themselves. 0.9999 of each atom is space, with only 0.0001 being matter, which is moving at the speed of light.

Since all energy and matter are variations of the same thing, is it possible that *spirit matter* is the energy phase of reality, and *physical matter* is the physical or element phase of reality? "There is no such thing as immaterial matter," Joseph Smith was told. "All spirit is matter, but it is more fine or pure, and can only be discerned by purer eyes."[11] Is the more fine and pure matter of the spirit just organized energy? If so, what we see, hear, smell, or touch with our senses would be the physical or particle form of reality. The "real world" of our senses would be the physical side of a two sided reality. With their new discoveries about light and matter, perhaps modern-day physicists have finally touched on the spirit side of reality—the universal spirit of God which is present throughout the universe. If so, their discoveries could help us understand our God and his gospel of light.

In the energy form, all elements have access to the whole universe. They are omnipresent. There is no center or local position, but any part is equal to the whole, allowing sub-atomic parts to be connected, and to communicate instantly. In the form of matter, what we see as individual parts, including people, are but the organized *physical* part of a larger universal *spiritual* whole. We are spiritually connected with all other parts in the universe, including with each other. One electron is no more independent from the universe than one cell is independent from the whole body.

UNITING TWO TRUTHS INTO ONE

Discovering that light is two things and not one, is the key to understanding our universe.[12] Truth has two faces, wave and particle, energy and matter, interconnected yet independent. Since God is the ultimate truth of the cosmos and since God is light, it is logical that he should be an expression of the two forms of truth. The mystery of God is the same mystery as the mystery of light, energy and matter—two seemingly different parts of one reality. God is a being connected to the entire universe, giving light and life to all elements and matter, understanding and feeling the sorrows and joys of billions of humans at the same moment. Yet, God is a separate individual with a glorified body, isolated in time and space.

Is God, with glorified flesh and bones, truth in its physical, particle form? Is God, omnipresent throughout the universe, truth as organized energy, in its spirit form? Is his spirit the interconnected, timeless part of light, and his glorified physical body of flesh and bones the other half of reality—the physical particle form, in time and place? If so, celestial life would mean having full access to both forms of reality. The veil we are within during mortal life would be our restriction to the physical form of reality, preventing us from coming into the universal spirit presence of God. In mortality our physical bodies are dominant over our spiritual bodies, unlike God, who would have equal and full access to both spirit and matter.

The experience of the brother of Jared supports the idea that there is a dual nature to God and to Christ. The brother of

Jared prepared stones to be placed in dark barges for light, thinking he would rely upon the graciousness of Christ to touch the stones to make them shine. He took the stones to a high mountain and petitioned Christ to touch them so they would give light. As the Lord touched the stones, the brother of Jared saw the finger of the Lord. "The Lord stretched forth his hand and touched the stones one by one with his finger. *And the veil was taken from off the eyes of the brother of Jared, and he saw the finger of the Lord.*"[13] The brother of Jared was struck with fear because he had never imagined the Lord would have a body. The Lord revealed his whole spiritual body to the brother of Jared and explained that his spiritual body was in the same form of his future physical body. The Lord then told the brother of Jared, "Because thou knowest these things ye are redeemed from the fall; therefore ye are brought back into my presence; therefore I show myself unto you."[14]

We are not surprised that God has a finger, because Joseph Smith taught us he does, but what we should ask is, "Where was the rest of the body of Christ when the brother of Jared saw only the finger?" In a universe with two forms of light and truth, the brother of Jared would have seen the finger of the Lord in its particle form but wouldn't have seen the remaining part of the Lord because it would be in the wave form. At first the veil was only separated no further than the joint of the finger. At that time the Lord was present in both forms of light, the finger in the particle form and the remaining part of his body in the wave form.

God's own intelligence was at one time organized with energy, the wave form of light, or what we would call spirit. He was again organized with matter, physical flesh, the particle form of reality. Having been resurrected into celestial glory, he became perfected pure light. Being in both forms of light he could have full power over all the elements in the universe, while retaining his refined body of flesh and bone, and he could declare to his earthly children, "Thus saith the Lord your God . . . the same which looked upon the wide expanse, and all the seraphic hosts of heaven, before the world was made; The same which knoweth all things, for all are present before mine eyes."[15]

Christians, as a whole, have concentrated only on the omnipresent form of God, discounting the possibility of a second form, which would allow God to have a physical body. Some Christians have categorized Mormons as non-Christian because of our insistence that God has a glorified physical body. Mormons have had difficulty explaining the dual nature of a God with physical parts on one hand and universal presence in the cosmos on the other. Interestingly our theology coincides with what scientists now know about the nature of light, especially since the scriptures repeatedly inform us that our God is light. Is the grand secret of the nature of God that he is both infinite and finite—the ultimate expression of matter, energy, and light? Is he both wave and particle, energy and matter, spirit and body, everywhere and somewhere, universal yet personal, all powerful yet intimate, the revelation of justice and the cradle of mercy?

Chapter 4
God and His Attributes

"I am the Almighty God" (Genesis 17:1)

The scriptures describe our God as having two opposite forms. He is both spirit and matter. He is everywhere and yet somewhere. It is not easy to accept facts which cannot be fully explained, or facts that seem contradictory. It is not easy to understand that our Father in Heaven has dual characteristics. But the scriptures and our prophets say God is infinite and finite. Since God is light and all the scientific evidence points to different traits of light and matter, we should expect God to be an expression of both facets of light. For all we know, God may have even more facets of light which we are not yet aware of.

In the Christian world, only Mormonism has taught that God is a finite glorified being with infinite attributes. We have held to our faith without understanding how he could be both, even concentrating on his finite qualities more than his infinite qualities. We have been scorned because we believe he is both. We have been told that we should abandon our belief that he is finite and accept him only as infinite. Philosophical and theological arguments about God have only centered on whether he is infinite or whether he is finite. But the nature of light and matter has taught us that reality is both infinite and finite. It is therefore reasonable to accept that God is both infinite and finite, instead of trying to make him one or the other.

THE INFINITE ATTRIBUTES OF GOD

In proclaiming himself the Almighty, God declares his perfection. There is none greater than he, and there is no power that transcends his light and glory. Light is the power by which he creates worlds without end.[1] His almighty power of light brings order out of chaos, structuring the elements to express his marvelous creations. He reveals his glory through his love, mercy, power, and knowledge—all expressions of his light. These are the essences of his attributes as we know them. To understand God is to understand his attributes which are his perfection. "What are we to understand by the perfections of Deity?" Joseph Smith asks in the 5th *Lecture on Faith,* and then answers, "The perfections which belong to his attributes." His perfect attributes influence all his "kingdoms" in the universe, including the kingdoms of intelligences, spirits, the elements and his mortal creations. Therefore whoever sees or feels "any or the least of these hath seen God moving in his majesty and power."[2]

THE OMNIPRESENCE OF GOD

It is in the spirit that God is everywhere. Even though he has a spirit body as we do, that spirit body could not possibly contain all of the spiritual light he has. Remember that visual light is only one small part of the electromagnetic spectrum. What we see is not all we get! Radiation energy from the sun includes much more than just what is visual. Where "the sun" begins and where it ends is not a black and white line. Why should it be any different with God? God's light in the spirit could be pure organized energy. It is infinite and omnipresent throughout the universe. It is not just God's influence which is everywhere, but God himself is everywhere. We cannot comprehend God's spirit any more than we can comprehend light in its wave form. We cannot comprehend his infinite character in mortality because we are veiled from his powerful light.

Since God's perfection includes his perfect light, there is no darkness in him, and his perfect light allows him to be present in all things. He is "the light which is in all things, which giveth life to all things . . . (He) is in the bosom of eternity, who is in the midst of all things."[3] His is the light which is intelligence,[4] and he is in the elements,[5] allowing him to be omnipresent. "God had material to organize the world out of chaos" Joseph Smith taught, "chaotic matter, which is element, and *in which dwells all the glory*."[6] God not only declared he "is above all things, and in all things, and is through all things," but revealed "I am the true light that is in you, and that you are in me; otherwise ye could not abound."[7] God's spiritual being is throughout the universe and it is his presence that maintains the universe.

Realizing that it is possible for God's spirit or energy to continually be in all things, at all times, makes statements like Orson Pratt's more understandable. Pratt wrote that God did not just construct the universe and then "step aside to see the mighty fabric operate. . . . *God is every moment in nature, and every moment acts upon nature, and through nature, the same as the spirit of man acts in, and through and upon the tabernacle of his body. If God should withdraw himself from nature, or should cease to act upon it, that portion of it without life or intelligence, (if there be any such portion) would immediately cease all action*: and while thus apart from nature no law could be given to it which could be obeyed: no gravitative or cohesive tendencies could be exerted upon it; no chemical combinations or organic operations could be performed; or in other words, unintelligent nature would be entirely dead, and no voice or power could awake it, or have the least effect upon it, without [God's presence] entering into it, and operating upon it, and through it."[8]

It is not just the present moment in which God fills the universe. His omnipresence includes all time, past, present and the future. "All things are present before mine eyes,"[9] God teaches, and "there is no God beside me, and all things are present with me, for I know them all,"[10] for the "past, present, and future, . . . are continually before the Lord."[11]

THE OMNISCIENCE OF GOD

"Intelligence, or the light of truth, was not created or made, neither indeed can be."[12] Because intelligence is truth and light, it is our eternal conscience. God said, "The glory of God is intelligence or, in other words, light and truth."[13] In other words, intelligence has the innate quality to know truth and light, because truth and light is its nature. God told Joseph Smith that truth is spirit,[14] and "truth is knowledge of things as they are, and as they were, and as they are to come."[15]

God's omnipresent energy of light can explain how he is omniscient. Alma declared, "The Spirit knoweth all things."[16] God declared to Israel, "I am God, and there is none else; I am God, and there is none like me, Declaring the end from the beginning, and from ancient times the things that are not yet done, saying, My counsel shall stand, and I will do all my pleasure."[17] Joseph Smith wrote, "God is . . . perfect intelligence, and . . . His wisdom is alone sufficient to govern and regulate the mighty creations and worlds."[18] In the *Lectures on Faith* Joseph Smith stated that without the knowledge of all things God would not be able to save any portion of his creature, and we would not be able to exercise faith in him.

When God's glory rested upon Moses, Moses experienced a portion of God's omniscience and beheld every particle of the earth, the inhabitants thereof, "and he discerned them by the Spirit of God; and their numbers were great, even numberless as the sand upon the sea shore. And he beheld many lands; and each land was called earth, and there were inhabitants on the face thereof."[19] After Moses comprehended more than he had ever imagined, God clarified that there was even more, but it was beyond what Moses could comprehend. "But only an account of this earth, and the inhabitants thereof, give I unto you. For behold, there are many worlds that have passed away by the word of my power. *And there are many that now stand, and innumerable are they unto man; but all things are numbered unto me, for they are mine and I know them.*"[20] After receiving a portion of God's glory and understanding, Moses "said unto himself: Now for this cause I know that man is nothing, which thing I never had supposed."[21] God's glory came upon Moses and the veil between the physical world and spiritual world was removed enough that he comprehended the omniscience of our Father. Because we are restricted to mortality, our minds are inadequate to comprehend an all-knowing, all-present, and all-powerful being without God's grace helping us rend the veil.

THE OMNIPOTENCE OF GOD

God reveals himself as a being of glory, light and power. "I am the almighty God,"[22] he declared. "Behold, and hearken unto the voice of him who has all power, who is from everlasting to everlasting, even Alpha and Omega, the beginning and the end."[23] God is "the light of the sun and the power thereof by which it was made," and he is also the light of the moon, the stars and the earth, and "the power by which they were made."[24] God is the power that gives life and law to all matter, whether animate or inanimate,[25] and therefore all things are dependent upon him. In Joseph Smith's words, "[T]here is a God, possessing all the attributes ascribed to Him by all Christians of all denominations; . . . He reigns over all things in heaven and on earth, and . . . all are subject to His power."[26]

God proclaimed that his light proceeds from his presence "to fill the immensity of space." His "light which is in all things" gives "life to all things." His light "is the law by which all things are governed, even the power of God. . . . All kingdoms have a law given; And there are many kingdoms; for there is no space in the which there is no kingdom; and there is no kingdom in which there is no space, either a greater or lesser kingdom. And unto every kingdom is given a law;

and unto every law there are certain bounds also and conditions."[27]

Where there is space, there is matter; and where there is matter, there is law; and where there is law, there is light. Thus, there is no space without light. Light, matter and law are ubiquitous expressions of God's power and presence. Lehi taught that if there were no law, there would be no God.[28] In a scientific sense, when God declares he is the power of creation, light and life, he is declaring that he is the law and the power of the universe. He is the fullness of light in all its forms.

God's power includes not just the creative genius to organize matter out of chaos and imbue each particle with his spirit, but his power also includes the promise that life and matter will be maintained forever, for God is eternal. It is this aspect of the power of God, the power to fulfill his word, which is most important to us. "But the Lord knoweth all things from the beginning; wherefore, he prepareth a way to accomplish all his works among the children of men; for behold he hath all power unto the fulfilling of all his words."[29] God's power includes the promise to bring us back into his bosom, as were the inhabitants of the City of Enoch.[30] "I know, O Lord," declared the brother of Jared, "that thou hast all power, and can do whatsoever thou wilt for the benefit of man,"[31] even "all power . . . to the destroying of Satan and his works at the end of the world."[32] Most importantly, in the words of Alma, God has "power to save every man that believeth on his name and bringeth forth fruit meet for repentance."[33]

It is in his power to fulfill all promises that God reveals the power of his love, mercy and justice. To know of his goodness and love is to comprehend his glory, [34] for "Glory, and honor, and power, and might, be ascribed to our God; for he is full of mercy, justice, grace and truth, and peace, forever and ever."[35] Man petitions God saying, "O Lord God Almighty, hear us in these our petitions, and answer us from heaven, thy holy habitation, where thou sittest enthroned, with glory, honor, power, majesty, might, dominion, truth, justice, judgment, mercy, and an infinity of fullness, from everlasting to everlasting."[36] And God answers by giving us his spirit and Comforter. "Therefore it is given to abide in you; the record of heaven; the Comforter; the peaceable things of immortal glory; the truth of all things; that which quickeneth all things, which maketh alive all things; that which knoweth all things, and hath all power according to wisdom, mercy, truth and justice and judgment."[37]

Since God is purified, perfect light, his omniscience, omnipotence, and omnipresence can all be explained through the spirit form of light—energy, allowing him to be infinite, timeless, filling the universe with perfect love, life, and mercy, and influencing all elements.

THE FINITE ATTRIBUTES OF AN INFINITE GOD

In the physical form of matter God exists in time and space with a glorified resurrected body of flesh and bones, eternally progressing, expressing love and mercy. God's light in the physical form can be compared to the particle form of light. Just as light is both wave and particle at the same moment, so should it be with God. Just as subatomic parts are energy and matter at the same moment, so should it be with God. He is not either infinite or finite, omnipresent or in space, in time or out of time, but he is all of these at the same moment. As mysterious as that sounds, there is real majesty here. God is whole, having united all aspects of reality by becoming the fullness of light in all its forms. He is not veiled from any aspect of reality, being present in all. He is perfect because he is perfect in all forms of light. Nothing could be more majestic.

TIME AND THE VEIL

In the spirit form of reality, where all things are infinite, everywhere present and interconnected, there would be no specific place of residence, no one locality, no center and no time. Everything is everywhere, with God in the midst of all things, past, present and future,[38] just as the scriptures and prophets say he is. But in the physical form of reality, there is space, and therefore, things are finite and in time. Time came into being for us when God organized space and matter out of energy, when he organized the physical phase of elements. It is God who has organized all the solar systems and has declared that their revolutions govern their times.[39] "He hath given a law unto all things, by which they move in their times and their seasons; And their courses are fixed, even the course of the heavens and the earth, which comprehend the earth and all the planets. And they give light to each other in their times and in their seasons, in their minutes, in their hours, in their days, in their weeks, in their months, in their years—all these are one year with God, but not with man."[40]

In other words, many "times" equal one "time" with God.[41] God is in all of the times and seasons at once. "Now whether there is more than one time appointed for men to rise it mattereth not; for all do not die at once, and this mattereth not; all is as one day with God, and time only is measured unto man."[42] Surely our Father has the agency and ability to choose in which of the many times throughout the universe he will appear in his physical form. When Jesus Christ and his Father came to Joseph Smith in the grove, they were finite beings, with glorified bodies, being in the time and in the space of this kingdom we call earth. Their wholeness would allow them not only to be omnipresent in the spirit, but their wholeness would also allow them to be in time, and to choose in which kingdom of time their finite bodies will reside at any given moment.

We are in time on this earth, but we will be without time when we return to our Heavenly Parents. The scriptures prophesy that after Satan is bound there will be no time. In clarifying the seven trumps as described by John the Revelator,[43] God teaches, "And so on, until the seventh angel shall sound his trump; and he shall stand forth upon the land and upon the sea, and swear in the name of him who sitteth upon the throne, that there shall be time no longer."[44] The veil of time is our restriction to the particle form of reality. "As quickly as the spirit is unlocked from this house of clay," Brigham Young taught, "it is free to travel with lightning speed to any planet, or fixed star, or to the uttermost part of the earth, or to the depths of the sea, according to the will of Him who dictates."[45] Elder Neal A. Maxwell reminds us:

> Eventually, the veil that now encloses us will be no more. Neither will time. (D&C 84:100) Time is clearly not our natural dimension. Thus it is that we are never really at home in time. Alternately, we find ourselves wishing to hasten the passage of time or to hold back the dawn. We can do neither, of course, but whereas the fish is at home in water, we are clearly not at home in time—because we belong to eternity. Time, as much as any one thing, whispers to us that we are strangers here.[46]

We are only half expressed, having come from the timeless presence of God and on the path to return there. Our inner drive is to be again united in our native state, with our Heavenly Parents, who are infinite, without time, and finite, in time.

THE ADDED GLORY OF GOD

God's work is "to bring to pass the immortality and eternal life of man," and what he receives for his work is glory or light.[47] God, who is perfect, can still progress by expanding his glory. Perfection and progression are not mutually exclusive concepts. Having perfect love does not mean God cannot experience additional joy from the love he gives. The nature of love is that it cannot be given without expanding itself. It is impossible to express love without receiving an increase of love back again. If "God is light,"[48] and "God is Love,"[49] light is love. Light moves out from itself to encompass others. In human terms, we call it love. In scriptural terms, it is also called joy.

When Nephi partook of the tree of life "it filled [his] soul with exceedingly great joy."[50] He learned that the tree's fruit represented Christ's atonement and therefore it was "the love of God."[51] The light of God's love infuses joy into us.[52] "It is the love of God which . . . is the most desirable above all things."[53] We receive joy by giving love. "How great will be your joy if you should bring many souls unto me."[54] Our Heavenly Parents, with perfect love, continue to progress in joy by giving their love and light to us. When we see a perfect sunset or receive a perfect embrace, it does not mean we have received all the joy there is. We continue to receive additional joy with each new sunset and each new embrace. God can feel perfect joy every time another person is willing to receive more light, more agency and more connectedness. With an infinite number of intelligences to give his love to, there is an infinite amount of light and joy that will be returned to him. Alma labored to bring other souls "to taste the exceeding joy which he [had] tasted."[55] Perhaps our Heavenly Parents renew themselves and progress by helping us experience what they have experienced.

The progression of God through increased joy could also include receiving joy by sacrificing. Our Father receives the passion of joy when we receive him,[56] and the passion of sorrow when we don't. While talking to Enoch, God wept when he saw the wickedness of men, that they would not "love one another."[57] Enoch didn't understand how a perfect God could weep. God taught Enoch the significance of sacrifice and mercy, and then Enoch wept also until God again told him of the atoning sacrifice of Christ. When Enoch felt the passion of God's love, "his heart swelled wide as eternity."[58] Giving light to others is paramount in the physical phase of reality, because it is in this life where opposites are fully revealed, allowing sacrifice its full expression. The atonement, which is the greatest manifestation of God's love, had to be accomplished in the flesh where there is opposition. (See 'CHRIST AND THE ATONEMENT' Chapter Nine, JESUS CHRIST: GOD OF LIGHT COMES TO EARTH)

Elder John A. Widtsoe said, "The Savior gave of Himself, gave His very life that we might live. To sacrifice that others might be blessed was His word, His work, His life. Sacrifice is the evidence of true love. Without sacrifice love is not manifest. Without sacrifice there is no real love and kindness. . . . We love no one unless we sacrifice for him. We can measure the degree of love that we possess for any man or cause, by the sacrifice we made for him, or it. . . . Sacrifice lifts us toward the likeness of God, the likeness of our Elder Brother Jesus Christ."[59]

We believe that God was once as we are now, separated from the universal light of his God. Our God had to at some time be glorified and accepted into the full light and glory of his own Heavenly Father. When that happened our God as a finite, glorified, physical man, must have gained access into the infinite spirit of all Gods before him and he must have received a fullness. All that his Father had was given to him, just as he has promised he will give us all he has.[60] The basic function of light is just one thing—to be given away. The way we receive more light is to give away the light we already have, the ultimate expression being the giving of life to gain life.[61] One way God receives added glory must be centered in receiving joy by giving love and knowledge to others. One way we progress is by receiving God's light and then giving it away as he would. By giving away light to immature intelligences, God must progress by helping them progress. His glory becomes our glory, progression and joy, and our glory becomes his glory, progression and joy, and in a real way we become one with him.

Chapter 5
Near-Death Experiences and God's Light

"The Lord lift up His countenance upon thee, and give thee peace" (Numbers 6:26)

Our spiritual roots come from the revelations of our prophets. What Moses learned in vision of the creation is what we have in the Book of Genesis. Nephi, like most early prophets, was endowed with light on a mountain top. Temples were built so the prophets' descendants would also be endowed with light. Each of us yearns for insight into our past spirit life and each of us feels anxious about our future life after death. We have passed down to us through family histories and journals the spiritual experiences and visions of our ancestors and we are edified from what they have learned and taught us. Those snapshots of past and future lives help form our concepts of the beauty of God and his kingdom.

Over the last twenty years men and women have become less afraid of expressing the spiritual aspects of their near-death experiences, the experience of being physically dead, then coming back to life. What is so exciting about near-death experiences is that thousands of ordinary people have had them. Each experience is individual but reveals universal truths of love and light. Their experiences break through the restriction of their physical bodies, giving them access to the ubiquitous spirit of God. Not only have near-death experiences changed the lives of those who have the experiences, but their experiences can touch our souls, teach us and bring us closer to living by the light of God.

Near-death experiences have shown a uniformity that supports their validity. Even though science cannot explain what happens, the evidence supports what Latter-day Saints know about life beyond this earth. One non-Mormon author, Raymond Moody, details in several pages in his book, *The Light Beyond*, the Mormon concept of the hereafter because near-death experiences often confirm the Mormon view of the other side of life.[1] There have been several books written specifically on the subject of near-death experiences and Mormonism.[2,3,4] Near-death experiences have been a course of study at Brigham Young University and in many medical schools. There is currently an international association for near-death studies which is dedicated to scientific research and understanding of near-death experiences.

BEINGS OF LIGHT

Just as light is central to prophetic visions, light in some form is universal to near-death experiences. People who have near-death experiences describe seeing beings of light and whole cities of light. The beings of light are brighter than anything on earth. Their brilliance doesn't hurt the eyes, but is warm, vibrant and alive and is associated with a feeling of total love and acceptance. The light "continued to increase in intensity until it seemed to be equal to a million welders' light. I knew if I had been seeing through my human eyes instead of those of my spiritual body I would have been blinded."[5]

The beauty and magnetism of the light is overwhelming. "I became aware of the most powerful, radiant light, brilliant white light. It totally absorbed my consciousness. It shone through this glorious scene like the sun rising on the horizon through a veil which had suddenly opened. This magnificent light seemed to be pouring through a brilliant crystal. It seemed to radiate from the very center of the consciousness I was in and to shine out in every direction through the infinite expanses of the universe. . . . Even though the light seemed thousands and thousands of times stronger than the brightest sunlight, it did not bother my eyes. My only desire was to have more and more of it and to bathe in it forever."[6] "These beings aren't composed of ordinary light. They glow with a beautiful and intense luminescence that seems to permeate everything and fill the person with love. . . . It's almost like being drenched by a rainstorm of light."[7]

Seeing and feeling the light beyond this life through near-death experiences reveal not just the power of God but our own immortal nature. "It was a dynamic light, not like a spotlight. It was an incredible energy—a light you wouldn't believe. I almost floated in it. It was feeding my consciousness feelings of unconditional love, complete safety and complete, total perfection . . . It just *powed* into you. My consciousness was going out and getting larger and taking in more; I expanded and more and more and more came in. It was such rapture, such bliss. And then, and then a piece of knowledge came in: it was that I was immortal, indestructible. I cannot be hurt, cannot be lost. We don't have anything to worry about. And that the world is perfect; everything that happens is part of a perfect plan. I don't understand this part now, but I still know it's true."[8]

Compare the edification of those who have near-death experiences with the wonderment of Oliver Cowdery, speaking about his spiritual experiences while with Joseph Smith. "These were days never to be forgotten—to sit under the sound of a voice dictated by the inspiration of heaven, awakened the utmost gratitude of this bosom! . . . On a sudden, as from the midst of eternity, the voice of the Redeemer spake peace to us, while the veil was parted and the angel of God came down clothed with glory, and delivered the anxiously looked for message, and the keys of the gospel of repentance. What joy! what wonder! what amazement! . . . Our eyes beheld, our ears heard, as in the 'blaze of day'; yes more—above the glitter of the May sunbeam, which then shed its brilliancy over the face of nature! Then his voice, though mild, pierced to the center and, his words, 'I am thy fellow-servant,' dispelled every fear. We listened, we gazed, we admired! 'Twas the voice of an angel from glory, 'twas a message from the Most High! And as we heard we rejoiced, while His love enkindled upon our souls, and we were wrapped in the vision of the Almighty! Where was room for doubt? Nowhere; uncertainty had fled, doubt had sunk no more to rise, while fiction and deception had fled forever!"[9]

In trying to describe what they saw and how it made them feel, those who have had near-death experiences express themselves much the same way Oliver did. Most say their experiences were so out of this world that they did not have the language to express the beauty and love they felt. And just like Moses, they understood that it was God's spirit upon them that allowed them to experience God's glorious light. Most described the light as love, mercy or peace, supporting our scriptures when they refer to the glory and love of God. "When I was embraced, I felt a warmth all through me. And there was a feeling of love. . . . it was like that was all the love there was, everything. It was like . . . I can't explain the feeling. It's beyond words."[10]

Those who have had a vision of God's glory while in the flesh have felt that same overwhelming feeling of love and lack of words to describe the experience. After Christ prayed for the Nephites, the scriptures say, "the things he prayed cannot be written," — not that they should not be written, but that the things heard and seen were beyond words to express. "The eye hath never seen, neither hath the ear heard, before, so great and marvelous things as we saw and heard Jesus speak unto the Father; And no tongue can speak, neither can there be written by any man, neither can the hearts of men conceive so great and marvelous things as we both saw and heard Jesus speak"[11]

The Nephites then had a vision of their children being tended by angels and encircled by the glory of God when "they saw the heavens open, and they saw angels descending out of heaven as it were *in the midst of fire*; and they came down and encircled those little ones about, and *they were encircled about with fire*; and the angels did minister unto them. And the multitude did see and hear and bear record . . . every man for himself."[12] The gospel of light is the promise of God's glorious light encircling us with purifying fire, cleansing us and lifting us again into his presence as glorified beings of light, as he is.

EXPERIENCING THE UNIVERSAL NATURE OF GOD

Those who have had near-death experiences and have broken through the veil into God's light have touched the *omnipresence* and *omniscience* of God. "The near-death experiencer has learned that past, present, and future are all simultaneously one to God, and that they have experienced the 'all present now' of God in their experience of the divine."[13] "There is, first of all, a sense of having total knowledge, but specifically one is aware of seeing the entirety of the earth's evolution and history, from the beginning to the end of time."[14]

"At one point I had complete knowledge of everything, from beginning of creation to the end of time."[15] "I had the feeling that I knew why things are as they are, why all the problems on the earth were as they were. . . . it was an overwhelming feeling of knowing."[16] "About this time I had an experience that I'll never forget. . . . a feeling of total, total knowledge without asking. It's like you and me sitting here, now, and wondering how far the universe expands, or . . . just questions we have on earth about the geography of the earth, craters, or anything. This feeling I had of total knowledge was just that, I knew everything without asking. It was an incredible feeling."[17]

"It seemed that all of a sudden , all knowledge—of all that had started from the very beginning, that would go on without end—that for a second I knew all the secrets of all ages, all the meaning of the universe, the stars, the moon—of everything. . . . It was in all forms of communication, sights, sounds, thoughts. It was any—and everything. It was as if there was nothing that wasn't known. All knowledge was there, not just of one field, but everything."[18]

Spirit and *matter* are seen as a variation of the same thing. "Underlying this conception of the relation between body and spirit was an assumption that matter and spirit exist on a continuum, differing in degree rather than in kind."[19] "[My being] felt as if it had a *density* to it, almost, but not a physical density—kind of like, I don't know, waves or something, I guess: Nothing really physical, almost as if it were charged, if you'd like to call it that. But it felt as if it had something to it."[20]

Time and *space* are experienced as having no boundaries. "You could say [my experience] lasted one second or that it lasted ten thousand years and it wouldn't make any difference how you put it."[21] "I found myself in a space, in a period of time, I would say, where all space and time was negated."[22] "Something was strange about time, too, in this world where rules about space and speed and solid mass were all suspended. I had lost all sense of whether an experience was taking a split second, or whether it was lasting for hours."[23]

EXPERIENCING THE INTIMATE NATURE OF GOD

The various manifestations of light the scriptures describe are also experienced by those who have had near-death experiences. Feelings of *peace* and *love* are usually experienced, but they are qualified as only the surface of what really was felt. The peace was not of this world but was an overwhelming, all-embracing feeling of love, mercy and non-judgment just as Christ said. "Peace I leave with you, my peace I give unto you: Not as the world giveth , give I unto you. Let not your heart be troubled, neither let it be afraid."[24]

"The reason why [Christ] . . . is love is that love is the vessel of everything heavenly—that is, of peace, intelligence, wisdom, and happiness. For love accepts any and all things suitable to it; it wants them, seeks them out, and soaks them in gladly, so to speak, from a desire constantly to be enriched and fulfilled with them. . . . Love emanating from the Lord is the vessel of heaven and of everything there."[25] "Love is the major impression I still retain. In heaven there is light, peace, music, beauty and joyful activity, but above all there is love and within this love I felt more truly alive than I have ever done before. . . . What the light communicates to you is a feeling of true, pure love. You experience this for the first time ever."[26] "Everyone was in a state of absolute compassion to everything else. . . . love was the major axiom that everyone automatically followed. . . . There was nothing but love. . . it just seemed like the real thing, just to feel this sense of total love in every direction. . . . There was the warmest, most wonderful love. Love all around me. . . . Forever—eternal love. Time meant nothing. Just being. Love. Pure love. Love."[27] "And now abideth faith, hope, charity, these three; but the greatest of these is charity."[28]

"I was amazed at the mercy, understanding and love given to me while in the Savior's presence. There was such total acceptance and love -- no condemnation whatsoever. Standing in His presence I received a new perception of myself and of my worth. I had left the earth thinking of myself as human garbage. In a few moments in His presence, and feeling for myself what he felt for me, I totally reevaluated my worth. I did matter; He did care. Even more than that - - he loved me, he forgave me. I was so overwhelmed by the utter love and peace and mercy that I did not want to leave."[29]

That Christ is glory and light is also supported by those who have seen him during near-death experiences. "Jesus was the light itself," not an abstraction, but "as much a 'person' as all the others. He was prophet, priest and king."[30] "I stared in astonishment as the brightness increased, coming from nowhere, seeming to shine everywhere at once. . . . It was impossibly bright. . . . And right in the middle of my amazement came a prosaic thought, . . . I'm glad I don't have physical eyes at this moment, . . . This light would destroy the retina in a tenth of a second. No, I corrected myself, not the light. He. He would be too bright to look at. For now I saw that it was not light but a Man who entered the room, or rather, a Man made out of light, though this seemed no more possible to my mind than the intensity of the brightness that made up His form."[31]

The more we learn from science, scriptures, prophets and all those who have touched the eternities through visions and near-death experiences, the more complete is our revelation of truth, and the clearer our view of the beauty of light. We are children of light, living in a universe organized of light in all its forms. We have experienced only a small portion of our God's amazing light, his universal power and connectedness, and his loving peace.

Part II

JESUS CHRIST HOLY GHOST

Chapter 6
Jesus Christ: Expression of the Father

"The Father and I are one" (D&C 93:3)

CHRIST'S LIGHT AND POWER IN THE SPIRIT WORLD

The life of Jesus Christ, from his role as the firstborn in the pre-mortal world, to his life on earth as the Only Begotten of the Father, to his return again unto his Father, is the revelation of how Jesus Christ came into the fullness of his Father's glory. Having assumed the Father's light, Christ became the expression of his Father. Christ's life is an epic tale of love, life and power. It is the revelation of a God who became the Son by making flesh his tabernacle so he might "dwell among the sons of men."[1] Christ's life shows a loving relationship with his Father united through truth and light which fill the universe. The scriptures tell a heroic tale of Jesus Christ, an elder brother assuming the full range of Godly light. In the pre-mortal world, Christ first assumed the light of his Father by cleaving to and comprehending the purity of his

Father's love from the very beginning, and thus he became one with God. Christ then clothed himself with physical elements and became the ultimate expression of light in the flesh, and thus gained full power of agency.

To measure any one specific wave length of light, a specific instrument must be used. We cannot use a radio to comprehend X-rays, nor can we see micro waves with our eyes. We have to obey the law of any given wave length if we wish to use its energy. There is no compromise here. Light is the fact and we make use of light only by becoming compatible with it. It is like music. Each individual tone is a wave with a particular wave length. Sound waves also have overtones, which are smaller units of the main wave. The first overtone of any given note is one octave above or below that note. Then there are sub-overtones such as a fifth, a fourth, and a third. The overtone vibrations are compatible with each other, because they are subsets of each other. Together overtones make beautiful music because their vibrations are compatible. We cannot make beautiful music by insisting that incompatible music tones make harmony. Music waves are what they are and we only create harmony by using compatible vibrations. It is the same with light waves. They are what they are. We don't change what is eternal. We can only comprehend what is. Eternal law is the fixed nature of light. We train our beings to be light-detecting instruments, vibrating with eternal light waves, making spiritual music, and comprehending what is by accepting light's eternal nature. We can become part of God's eternal light by understanding light's fixed nature and by accepting its healing warmth.

First and most important in the growth of Jesus was his attitude of obedience to what was eternal, the will and glory of his Father.² Christ's first act recorded in scripture was his subjugation to the plan and will of his Father. In the pre-mortal world, after Satan presented an alternate plan for the salvation of men, God said, "But, behold, my Beloved and Chosen from the beginning, said unto me—Father, *thy will be done*, and the glory be thine forever."³ Christ reinforced that he was obedient to his Father's will when he told the Nephites, "[I] have glorified the Father in taking upon me the sins of the world, in the which I have suffered the will of the Father in all things from the beginning."⁴ Christ took his first step in assuming light by becoming subject to truth, the will of his Father, which allowed Christ to become the first of God's spirit children to obtain the fullness of God's glory. Christ's obedience also positioned him to become our Savior, a place of honor, to deliver to us the same fullness of light which he had received.

"I will make him my firstborn, higher than the kings of the earth,"⁵ the Psalmist has said. Being the firstborn in the spirit means being the first intelligence of light to be clothed with spirit matter. Christ subsequently became the most intelligent of all the spirits who were born into the pre-mortal family of God. Christ told Abraham, "These two facts do exist, that there are two spirits, one being more intelligent than the other; there shall be another more intelligent than they; *I am the Lord thy God, I am more intelligent than they all.*"⁶ Since knowledge and intelligence are light, this scripture is also saying God has more light than all others. Not just more intelligent or more light than the second most intelligent spirit, but more intelligent and light than all other spirits added together.

Christ began to assume eternal glory when he was born with a spirit body of light. He revealed himself in that spirit form to the brother of Jared and said, "Behold, this body, which ye now behold, is the body of my spirit; and man have I created after the body of my spirit; and even as I appear unto thee to be in the spirit will I appear unto my people in the flesh."[7] The Father's plan is not only to clothe his firstborn son with his light and glory, but to do the same with all his spirit children. That plan for us was based on the same basic law that Christ accepted, obedience to light and truth. That plan, according to Elder Bruce R. McConkie, "called for one of Deity's spirit sons to be born into mortality as the Only Begotten in the flesh, who would thus inherit from the Father the power of immortality; it called for this Chosen One to work out an infinite and eternal atonement whereby fallen men would be raised in immortality, while those who believed and obeyed would gain eternal life."[8]

When Christ, in obedience, said to his Father, "Father, thy will be done, and the glory be thine forever,"[9] Christ accepted all the conditions of that plan, including his own future sacrifice. He then became "the lamb slain from the foundation of the world,"[10] and "the author of eternal salvation unto all them that obey him,"[11] just as he had obeyed his Father. It was in preparation for his future sacrifice that Christ assumed light, the attributes of his Father, and thus became like God. "There stood one among them," Abraham saw, "that was like unto God."[12] Christ stated he had glory from his Father, prior to coming to earth,[13] being the "Only begotten Son, who was in the bosom of the Father, even from the beginning."[14]

In the pre-earth life Christ assumed enough light to be one with his Father, part of the Godhead, with power to act in the capacity of a god. "All power is given unto me," Christ said, "in heaven and in earth."[15] Christ declared to Joseph Smith that He was the second Comforter, *"even the glory of the celestial kingdom; Which glory is . . . through Jesus Christ. . . .* He that ascended up on high, as also he descended below all things, in that he comprehended all things, that he might be in all and through all things, the light of truth."[16]

CHRIST EXPRESSES THE GLORY AND LIGHT OF THE FATHER

The Father's light and glory cannot be separated from him and he remain whole, any more than his hand could be removed and he remain whole. His spirit being of light is larger than his physical body. He is a glorified person with body and flesh, with full agency. Yet his spirit being of light extends beyond the bounds of that material body, so it can give light and life into every element of the universe. Since Christ assumed his Father's light by sharing the Father's glory in the pre-earth life, the oneness of Christ and his Father is not only oneness in purpose, but oneness in their shared light. They both are everywhere present in the energy phase of light, and therefore they are a common being in the spirit, yet they remain separate in the physical form of body and flesh. Since God the Father is everywhere present, and has all light and glory in the universe—past, present and future—it is reasonable that any person, Christ or otherwise, who gains the whole of our Father's light must become part of him.

The mystery here is how two beings can be one and still remain separate. It is similar to the mystery of how God can be both infinite and finite. It is also similar to the mystery of how light can be both wave and particle, everywhere and yet somewhere. Like the scientists who finally had to just accept light as it is, the solution to the mysteries of God, is to accept that there are two forms of truth. Just as light has two opposite forms, so do we, and so do God and Christ.

John declared the connectedness of the Father and the Son, that the Father dwells within the Son. "And I, John, bear record that [Christ] received a fulness of the glory of the Father: And [Christ] received all power, both in heaven and on earth, and the glory of *the Father was with him, for [the Father] dwelt in him.*"[17] Christ's own teachings reinforce his common being with his Father. "All things are delivered to me of my Father; and no man knoweth that the Son is the Father, and the Father is the Son, but him to whom the Son will reveal it."[18] To Phillip who asked Christ to show the Father, Christ said, "Believest thou not that I am in the Father, and the Father in me? the words that I speak unto you I speak not of myself: but the Father that dwelleth in me, he doeth the works. *Believe me that I am in the Father, and the Father in me*: or else believe me for the very works' sake."[19]

"Believe me that I am in the Father, and the Father in me." It is not a question. It is a declaration. "Believe me! And if you can't believe me because I say it, then believe me because of the works you have seen me do." Christ clarified to Joseph Smith the two parts of his being, Father and Son. "I am in the Father, and the Father in me, and the Father and I are one—The Father, because he gave me of his fulness, and the Son because I was in the world and made flesh my tabernacle, and dwelt among the sons of men."[20] In the physical form of elements, Christ is flesh, an individual with agency, but in the spirit form of light he is one with the Father, because they literally share common light.

In our pre-mortal life, God the Father already had a glorified body of flesh and bones. Christ did not. Christ shared the light and glory of his Father to the extent that Christ was designated God and Father.[21] There was a need for a god to come to earth for the salvation of the Father's other spirit children. Our heavenly Father, having a body already, chose Christ to descend to earth as God to save us. Thus Christ is the Son because he was obedient to his Father's wishes and took upon himself mortality. Christ is the Son because in the flesh, as in the pre-earth life, he became subject to his Father's will, including his Father's will that he suffer the indignities of mortals.

Because of the dual nature of Christ, there are some revelations in which he speaks as both the Father and the Son. It is as if Christ is revealing the light of both the Father and the Son and clarifying their oneness. To Joseph Smith, Christ said, "Listen to the voice of Jesus Christ, your Redeemer, the Great I Am." Near the end of the same revelation Christ says as the Father, "I, the Lord God, should send forth angels to declare unto them repentance and redemption through faith on the name of mine Only Begotten Son."[22]

On another occasion, the sequence is turned around where Christ begins the revelation speaking as the Father. "Thus saith the Lord; for I am God, and have sent mine Only Begotten Son into the world . . . and have decreed that he that receiveth him shall be saved, and he that receiveth him not shall be damned." In the closing of the same revelation Christ speaks as the Son. "Behold, I am Jesus Christ, and I come quickly. Even so Amen."[23]

The two roles of Christ, being both the Father and the Son, reveal the full unity of the Godhead, supporting how both glorified beings are of "the same divine mind, the same wisdom, glory, power, and fullness—filling all in all; the Son being filled with the fullness of the mind, glory, and power; or, in other words, the Spirit, glory, and power, of the Father, possessing all knowledge and glory, and in the same kingdom, sitting at the right hand of power, in the express image and likeness of the Father, mediator for man, being filled with the fullness of the mind of the Father; or in other words, the Spirit of the Father."[24]

CHRIST IS THE FATHER OF LIGHT TO MANKIND

Since our heavenly Father's powers are centered in Christ, what Christ gives to us is the Father's light and glory. There is a broad spectrum of the Father's light which includes not only all spiritual light but also physical light, including matter and electromagnetism. Our Father's glory of the Celestial kingdom comes through Christ, and Christ is the divine spirit that is in and through all things. It is the Father's light in Christ which is the light of the Sun, which "is the same light that quickeneth [our] understanding."[25] Visual light is Christ's light as much so as the light which touches our heart.

The light of Christ is the glory of God; it stretches across the same broad spectrum of visual and nonvisual planes. Christ's light "constitutes instinct in animal life," states Parley P. Pratt. "This is the true light which in some measure illuminates all men. . . . It is also in its higher degrees the intellectual light of our inward and spiritual organs, by which we reason, discern, judge, compare, comprehend, and remember the subjects within our reach. Its inspiration constitutes . . . reason in man."[26] These vital functions come from and are maintained by Christ's light or we "could not abound."[27]

We need the Spirit of Christ not only to help us discern the words of God,[28] but to help us with all powers of intellect. "We need the influence of the Spirit of God to quicken the light that is within us, for light cleaves to light, and the Spirit of God is light, and it cleaves unto the light that enters into the composition of the spirit of man; and when we keep his commandments the Lord is ever ready and willing to quicken the judgment, inform the mind, and lead us along in our thinking and reflecting powers, that we may have power to understand a great many truths."[29]

The same spirit that gives us understanding, also leads us in the direction of God. "For the word of the Lord is truth, and whatsoever is truth is light . . . even the Spirit of Jesus Christ. And the Spirit giveth light to every man that cometh into the world; and the Spirit enlighteneth every man through the world, that hearkeneth to the voice of the Spirit."[30] Through the light of Christ, what our minds think can lead us to what our hearts may feel. We "put [our] trust in that Spirit which leadeth to do good—yea, to do justly, to walk humbly, to judge righteously; and this is my Spirit. Verily, verily, I say unto you, I will impart unto you of my Spirit, which shall enlighten your mind, which shall fill your soul with joy."[31]

The light of Christ is the beacon call to all those who have already been touched by it through their desires to live good lives. Their enlightened minds and consciences connect them to the expanded light of the gospel. They find basic truth which then expands their understanding and directs them to the Spirit of Christ. Speaking of Jehovah, Brigham Young taught that, "God is the source, the fountain of all intelligence, no matter who possesses it, whether man upon the earth, the spirits in the spirit-world, the angels that dwell in the eternities of the Gods, or the most inferior intelligence among the devils in hell. All have derived what intelligence, light, power, and existence they have from God—from the same source from which we have received ours."[32]

There is also new spiritual life that Christ's light gives. The salvation that is provided through the light of Christ does not end with providing physical life. There is a new eternal life, a celestial life that is available to us by Christ finding his seed, creating a new family with his sons and his daughters. Through Christ's light we gain eternal life and become part of his family. "I am the Father and the Son," Christ declared to the brother of Jared. "In me shall all mankind have life, and that eternally, even they who shall believe on my name; *and they shall become my sons and my daughters.*"[33] We become the sons and daughters of Christ through accepting the atonement. The atonement is the passion of Christ in giving away all the glory and light he had accumulated. His atonement would glorify his Father by lifting us into the light of the celestial kingdom, to be with all immortal and eternal beings. (See "CHRIST AND THE ATONEMENT," Chapter nine, JESUS CHRIST: GOD OF LIGHT COMES TO EARTH)

By being obedient, Christ received all the glory and the power from his Father to create the heavens and the earth. Christ is therefore a reflection of the light of his Father.[34] Having assumed the glory of his Father, Christ placed himself between the Father and us. In doing so, Christ became the Father unto all humankind. He became, in all aspects, the revelation of his Father's glory and light. Christ is the Creator, the giver of life and light; the Great I Am, the Jehovah of the Old Testament; a babe laid in a manger, a King pinned upon a cross; our God in the flesh, our God the Redeemer; the light of the eye, the light of the soul; the essence of humility, the magnification of love; the strength of spirituality in the flesh, the full power of Savior in the resurrection; the unchanging hand of truth and judgment, the cradle of mercy and compassion. In all ways, Christ's light and glory is the Father's light and glory!

Chapter 7
Holy Ghost: Dispenser of Light

"The Holy Ghost beareth record of the Father and me"
(3 Nephi 28:11)

HOLY GHOST: MEMBER OF THE GODHEAD

Joseph Smith taught that there are three Gods in the Godhead: God the Father, God the Son and, "God the third, the witness or Testator."[1] The three "*is* one Eternal God,"[2] because they share the common light and glory of the Father. They are one in the spirit form of light since God the Father is the source of all light and glory in the universe and any being who shares that light becomes part of him. Christ became part of the Godhead by assuming the light of his Father. The Holy Ghost is one with the Father and Christ because his light is their light. In their physical form, the tangible form of elements, "The Father has a body of flesh and bones as tangible as man's; the Son also."[3] As a physical being, Christ is separate from his Father. Christ said he is *the*

Father "because [the Father] gave me of his fulness," yet Christ is *the* "*Son* because I was in the world and made flesh my tabernacle, and dwelt among the sons of men."[4] As individual physical beings, the Father and the Son have different roles to play, but they use their shared light to perform their individual roles.

The Holy Ghost uses that same light in his function as God the Testator. The Holy Ghost's role requires that he not have a physical body at this time so that he may personally touch the spirit form of our beings in bearing witness of Christ and his Father. "The Holy Ghost has not a body of flesh and bones, but is a personage of Spirit. Were it not so, the Holy Ghost could not dwell in us."[5]

HOLY GHOST: WITNESS OF THE FATHER AND SON

The Son has born witness of himself,[6,7] but there is not a scripture where the Holy Ghost bears witness of himself. "The Holy Ghost fell upon" Adam and "beareth record of the Father and the Son."[8] Our Father has given us the Holy Ghost to testify of Jesus Christ[9] for "no man can say that Jesus is the Lord, but by the Holy Ghost."[10] Jacob taught that it was by "the power of the Holy Ghost" that all the prophets wrote and prophesied of Christ. They learned by the Holy Ghost that "if there should be no atonement made all mankind must be lost."[11] "The Holy Ghost . . . beareth record of the Father and the Son; Which Father, Son and Holy Ghost are one God, infinite and eternal, without end."[12]

Christ told his disciples, "But when the Comforter is come, whom I will send unto you from the Father, even the Spirit of truth, which proceedeth from the Father, he shall testify of me."[13] What is it that the Comforter is going to bring from the Father, when he testifies of Christ? "Howbeit when he, the Spirit of truth, is come, he will guide you into all truth: for he shall not speak of himself; but whatsoever he shall hear, that shall he speak: and he will shew you things to come. He shall glorify me: *for he shall receive of mine, and shall shew it unto you.*"[14] The Holy Ghost receives what is the Father's and what is the Son's, and delivers it unto us. Since the Holy Ghost is the Testator of their God-ship, he must be delivering light and truth for light and truth are what makes them Gods.[15] Here again is another example of the basic operation of light, moving away from its original source. Apparently God and Christ have assigned the Holy Ghost to accelerate the give-away of their light. The faster light is given away, the more they are glorified in return. Christ has shown us through the paradox of the atonement that the very essence of the gospel of light is that by giving away everything, he received more back and in this way continued to progress and to be glorified.

HOLY GHOST: SPIRIT OF TRUTH

Since light is truth,[16] it is reasonable that both Christ and the Holy Ghost are called the Spirit of Truth. "I am the Spirit of Truth," Christ told Joseph Smith.[17] "My voice is Spirit; my Spirit is Truth; truth abideth and hath no end."[18] However, since Christ and the Holy Ghost share the same light, both are labeled the Spirit of Truth.

Just as there are different names given to the individual forms of light energy along the electromagnetic spectrum, there are different names given to the individual light qualities of the Holy Ghost. The Holy Ghost is called the "Comforter, . . . the Spirit of truth; whom the world cannot receive."[19] "When [the Holy Ghost], the Spirit of truth, is come, he will guide [us] into all truth."[20] Christ and the Holy Ghost are both called the Spirit of Truth, just as Christ and God the Father are both called Father. The relationship of Christ and the Holy Ghost is the same as the relationship of Christ and his Father. Christ is the Father because he has the same light as the Father. The Holy Ghost is the Spirit of Truth because he has the same Truth as Christ. Just as Christ received light and truth from the Father, the Holy Ghost receives light and truth from Christ. Therefore, what we receive from the Holy Ghost is not only a witness of Christ, but a witness of the Father.

The Holy Ghost is also called the Spirit of the Lord, a synonym for truth or light. "The Holy Ghost is the Spirit of the Lord, and issues forth from Himself, and may properly be called God's minister to execute His will in immensity; being called to govern by His influence and power."[21] The Spirit of the Lord Brigham Young talks about here is not the Spirit of Christ which is in the form of a man,[22] but is the light of Christ: Truth that has always existed, which fills the universe, governing all kingdoms.[23] When the Holy Ghost reveals the light of Christ to each of us individually, we receive revelation and are then opened to receive higher truths. "No man can receive the Holy Ghost without receiving revelations," Joseph Smith taught. "The Holy Ghost is a Revelator."[24] The Holy Ghost is a powerful magnifier of truth, concentrating light into those who ask "with a sincere heart, with real intent, having faith in Christ. . . . And by the power of the Holy Ghost [we] may know the truth of all things,"[25] "for the Comforter knoweth all things."[26]

The Holy Ghost takes light in its ubiquitous spirit form and centers it into our souls. Restricted by our physical mortal bodies, we need the Holy Ghost to direct holy light into us. He is a magnifier of light, a director of truth, and transmitter of all things from God and Christ to us.[27] When the Holy Ghost touches our spirits, he directs what we shall do and where we shall go,[28] what we preach,[29] and what we teach.[30] He makes known to us things from on high,[31] teaches us the truth and the way,[32] gives us the gospel in our own tongue,[33] and unfolds the mysteries of the kingdom through revelation.[34] He helps "set in order the churches," and helps us "study and learn, and become acquainted with all good books, and with languages, tongues, and people."[35] He reveals all truth that exists throughout the universe, and teaches us in both our hearts and our minds, for "this is the spirit of revelation."[36]

THE GIFT OF THE HOLY GHOST

The Holy Ghost reveals more than just the general truths of light. There are higher truths which require the personage of the Holy Ghost to continually "dwell in us."[37] Just like there are different energy levels along the electromagnetic spectrum of light, there should be different spirit energy levels that the Holy Ghost is in charge of. Perhaps the gifts of the Holy Ghost are the higher energy levels of the spirit. We need the presence of the Holy Ghost to gain wisdom and understanding,[38] power,[39] prophecy and visions,[40] and knowledge,[41] and to show signs, wonders, and miracles.[42] The Holy Ghost helps us speak in tongues,[43] brings all things to our remembrance,[44] including remembrance of Christ,[45] and most importantly, he shows us all things, including "the peaceable things of the kingdom."[46] Joseph Smith taught:

> There is a difference between the Holy Ghost and the gift of the Holy Ghost. Cornelius received the Holy Ghost before he was baptized, which was the convincing power of God unto him of the truth of the Gospel, but he could not receive the gift of the Holy Ghost until after he was baptized. Had he not taken this sign or ordinance upon him, the Holy Ghost which convinced him of the truth of God, would have left him. Until he obeyed these ordinances and received the gift of the Holy Ghost, by the laying on of hands, according to the order of God, he could not have healed the sick or commanded an evil spirit to come out of a man, and it obey him.[47]

Rights to this higher power of light of the Holy Ghost come only after we receive the testimony of Jesus Christ and after we are "baptized by water, and . . . receive the Holy

Ghost by the laying on hands, even as the apostles of old."[48] Christ taught Nicodemus, "Except a man be born of the water and the Spirit, he cannot enter into the kingdom of God."[49] Being brought into the light of Christ through the gift of spirit baptism means "being sanctified by the Holy Ghost,"[50] which allows us to "stand spotless before [Christ] at the last day."[51] Receiving spirit baptism is the visitation "with fire and with the Holy Ghost,"[52] bringing joy, a remission of sins, and peace of conscience.[53] Spirit baptism is the purifying fire promised by John the Baptist.[54] It is becoming spotless so we may "dwell with everlasting burnings."[55] It is having the personage of the Holy Ghost come upon us and dwell within us, bringing the light of God; cleansing our thoughts, our spirits and our bodies, fashioning us into beings of light like unto our Father and his Son. (See chapter fourteen, CHILDREN OF LIGHT: BECOMING GODS OF LIGHT)

Chapter 8
Creation: The Ordering of Light

"The Heavens declare the glory of God" (Psalm 19:1)

The creation, from both a scientific view and a religious view, is the light show of the cosmos. It is the pivotal act that opens the door between the two faces of light. It is the centerpiece of our existence, because it a major step which allows our two halves of reality, spirit and body, to join together as one whole. The creation story, from both a scientific side and a religious side, is exciting because the stories end the same—man is created—but the tales are told from completely different views. Both stories of the creation are the tales of how chaos became ordered, producing light, matter and life. Only the details are different.

THE BIG BANG

The most accepted theory among scientists about how our universe started is called the "big bang" theory. In the 1920s Edwin Hubble (the Hubble telescope orbiting the earth is named after him) spent three decades measuring the distances from the earth to other galaxies. He discovered that all the galaxies are moving away from ours, and the further away the galaxy is, the faster it is moving away. The galaxies in the universe are like raisins in leavened bread. As the bread raises, all the raisins continue to separate from each other. If we know how fast the galaxies are moving apart, and then calculate backwards, we come up with the age of the universe. According to the "big bang" theory, the whole universe started about 15 billion years ago from an infinitesimal speck that exploded, expanding to become all of the space, time, matter, and light which we now know as our universe. Current scientific evidence supports the theory that the universe started with a big bang and will continue to expand forever.

During the earliest stage of the universe, seconds after the big bang, there was complete chaos. The temperature of the cosmos was 10 million, billion, billion degrees (10 to the 32nd power) times hotter than the temperature at the center of our sun. It was so hot that photons, the particle stage of light, were knocking each other out of and into existence. Energy and matter were in a fluid stage and disorganized, quickly moving from matter to energy and back again. However, the energy phase was so strong that there was very little matter and therefore there was no organization to the matter that did exist. All parts of matter, from the nuclear sub-parts, to the electrons, were not only broken apart but were compressed by heat and gravity, keeping most in their energy form. It was like taking something apart into its tiniest components and then burning the components. What existed was unorganized light, a soup of electrons, matter and energy all mixed together in an unrecognizable glob.

The Bible calls the initial chaotic state of the universe a void, and says "the earth was without form, and void; and darkness was upon the face of the deep. And the Spirit of God moved upon the face of the waters."[1] After the big bang, there was a tremendous amount of light energy, but it was a dark energy because the temperature was so hot electrons could not stay in stable orbits to release visual light. As the universe expanded and gravity became dominant, solar systems began to form. When the temperature of the universe became cool enough (3000 degrees Kelvin) electrons could move into orbits around nuclei, and there release photons into space creating light. The religious side of the stories states, "And God said, Let there be light: and there was light. And God saw the light, that it was good: and God divided the light from the darkness."[2]

In the first two acts of creation—God's spirit moving upon the face of the water, and God commanding light to come forth—God separated the universe into opposites and withdrew light from the void, leaving the darkness. "I form the light, and create darkness."[3] "And they divided the light, or caused it to be divided, from the darkness."[4] It was the beginning of ordered light, creating the physical earth which would become the dominant learning ground for us in our physical phase. (The completion of the separation of all things would culminate in the garden of Eden when Adam and Eve fell, and the ultimate of opposites, life and death, came into existence.)

As the temperature of the universe continued to cool, matter, mainly hydrogen and helium, began to form from energy. Galaxies came into and out of existence. The elements were destroyed, created, destroyed and created again and again, billions of times. The scriptures says, "For behold, there are many worlds that have passed away by the word of my power. And there are many that now stand, and innumerable are they unto man; but all things are numbered unto me, for they are mine and I know them. . . . And as one earth shall pass away, and the heavens thereof even so shall another come; and there is no end to my works, neither to my words."[5] With insight far beyond his time, Orson Pratt wrote over a hundred years ago:

> *As the elements of all worlds were not created, but are eternal*, and as they have always been the tabernacle or dwelling place of God, *they must have eternally been acted upon by His Spirit; consequently must have passed through an endless series of operations without beginning.* . . . But this event was sudden, not the effects of slow and imperceptible changes, operating for an indefinite number of ages—*Jehovah spake—the elements came rushing together, not by their own power, but under the action of the self-moving forces of His Spirit, associated with the particles to be moved.* . . . [Philosophers] *would have called it the law of gravitation: while those better acquainted with the origin of the force would have called it the law by which the Spirit of God moves together the particles of matter.*[6]

GOD NOT A NEOPHYTE

Orson Pratt clarified the importance of remembering that it was the power of God which moved the elements together. The energy to organize the universe came out of God, just as light came out of God, just as light came out of Christ when the faithful woman touched his clothes and Christ felt virtue leave.[7] God is no stranger to the creation process. This universe is not his first experience. He has declared that "worlds without number have I created; and I also created them for mine own purpose. . . . And as one earth shall pass away, and the heavens thereof even so shall another come; and there is no end to my works, neither to my words."[8] The new physics would support the idea that there have been innumerable worlds which have come and gone.

Both science, scriptures and prophets support the idea that there was no creation out of nothing —ex nihilo. Not only has God always existed, but intelligence, matter, energy and light have also existed, co-eternal with God.[9,10] God told Joseph Smith, "Man was also in the beginning with God. Intelligence, or the light of truth, was not created or made, neither indeed can be. . . .For man is spirit. The elements are eternal, and spirit and element, inseparably connected, receive a fullness of joy."[11] B. H. Roberts wrote:

> Creation is not a bringing forth of something from nothing, but a transmutation of one substance into another form. . . . Creation, therefore, with those who accept the eternal existence—and therefore the co-eternal existence—of matter, force, and mind, can only regard 'creation' as events or changes wrought in an eternal universe. 'Creation' thus conceived, while it would never mean 'create' in the sense of bringing into existence force or matter or mind (spirit), yet it might be conceived of as bringing into new relations matter and force; and bring into existence new combinations, which really bring into being new things or new conditions.[12]

Since the universe was organized out of intelligence and matter, with energy which had always existed, perhaps what scientists call the "big bang" was just a re-organization of eternal elements, through the energy we call the power of God. Joseph Smith taught, "Now, the word create came from the word *baurau*, which does not mean to create out of nothing; it means to organize; the same as a man would organize materials and build a ship. Hence, we infer that *God had materials to organize the world out of chaos—chaotic matter, which is element, and in which dwells all the glory.*"[13]

In Abraham's account of the creation, "the Gods organized and formed the heaven and the earth."[14] The Gods then used their power to organize matter: "And the Gods ordered the expanse."[15] They not only ordered the expanse but, "the Gods watched those things which they had ordered until they obeyed."[16] There is a sequence here that recurs. The Lord organized matter by ordering some action. He then watched to see if there was obedience. "And the Gods said: We will do everything that we have said, and organize them; and behold, they shall be very obedient."[17] God then declared "that it was good," and after he had completed all his work, he declared "it was very good."[18] At the end of each creative period the scriptures declare, "And it came to pass that it was from evening until morning they called night; and it came to pass that it was from morning until evening that they called day."[19] The sequence of evening to morning is important in describing the ordering of chaos into our physical earth. There is a deeper meaning to the words "evening" and "morning" which clarifies the daily sequence of creation.

The Hebrew word for 'evening' is *erev*. This is the literal meaning of the word, although the root of *erev* carries with it implications far beyond that of a setting Sun. What is the visual sensation of evening? Darkness begins. Objects become obscure, blurred. The root of *erev* means just that, 'mixed up, stirred together, disorderly.' The Hebrew for 'morning' is *boker*. Its meaning is quite the opposite of *erev*. Morning brings the first light. Objects, visually mingled by dark of night, become distinct entities and this is the root meaning of *boker*, 'discernible, able to be distinguished, orderly'[20]

Each sequence ends with a declaration of opposites. There was disorder first and then there was order. It would make no sense if the Bible had read, "and there was morning and there was evening," because the couplet is really a declaration of what had just happened; disorder moved to order and darkness gave way to light. God used his power to separate the elements from energy and made sure the elements obeyed. God used his power to separate light into its two forms, wave and particle, by first organizing all things spiritually, and then by organizing all things physically.[21] He used his power to organize light into ordered energy and then to ordered elements. He used his power so we might experience the full range of the particle form of reality, the physical world. He used his power to separate the opposites of good and evil, so we could expand our agency to its full power.

The two tales of the creation from science and religion also support each other as to a variation of time throughout the universe. Prior to this century, time was thought to be absolute, flowing consistently at the same rate throughout the universe.

All events, regardless of where in the universe they were measured, were thought to occur at the same rate of time. In Sir Isaac Newton's words of three centuries ago, "Absolute, true and mathematical time, of itself, and from its own nature, flows equably without relation to anything external."[22]

The new physics have shown us that time is not constant throughout the cosmos. Time varies according to how fast a planet or solar system is traveling and how much gravity is present.[23] That means that when compared to each other, the time in one solar system could be millions of time faster or slower than the time in another solar system. That also means that it is impossible for one single clock to have timed all the events of the creation of the universe. There are billions of clocks keeping their own time, differing relative to each other, but all constant relative to their own time frame.

The scriptures support the variation of time throughout the universe. God has declared, "And again, verily I say unto you, he hath given a law unto all things, by which they move *in their time and their seasons*; And their courses are fixed, even the courses of the heavens and the earth, which comprehend the earth and all the planets. And they give light to each other *in their times and in their seasons,* in their minutes, in their hours, in their days, in their weeks, in their months, in their years—all these are one year with God, but not with man."[24]

Abraham was taught that there is a difference in time on the earth, moon and sun. "*Now the set time of the lesser light is a longer time as to its reckoning than the reckoning of the time of the earth upon which thou standest.* And where these two facts exist, there shall be another fact above them, that is, there shall be another planet whose reckoning of time shall be longer still; And thus *there shall be the reckoning of the time of one planet above another*, until thou come nigh unto Kolob, which Kolob is after the reckoning of the Lord's time. . . . And it is given unto thee to know the set time of all the stars that are set to give light, until thou come near unto the throne of God."[25]

One way to resolve the conflict between the scientific age and religious age of the earth is to accept that the earth has been on two time clocks: one clock when it was with God and in his reference frame of six days, and a second clock for the known age of the universe of 15 billion years as seen from our current reference frame. Did something happen to change reference frames from God's time to our current time? Abraham saw Adam and Eve in the Garden of Eden before they had tasted of the fruit of the tree of knowledge of good and evil, and saw that their time was after the Lord's time. "Now I, Abraham, saw that [the earth] was after the Lord's time, which was after the time of Kolob; for as yet the Gods had not appointed unto Adam his reckoning."[26]

Apparently the earth was still on God's time until Adam and Eve fell and then their reckoning of time began, which is the current clock from which we mark time. John Taylor taught that at the transgression of Adam the earth fell "from where it was organized, near the planet Kolob."[27] The early church publication, *Times and Seasons*, states that after the fall, "the earth no longer retained its standing in the presence of Jehovah; but was hurled into the immensity of space. . . . when [Adam] fell from the presence of the Lord the whole of his dominion fell also."[28] If the fall of Adam and Eve precipitated a time change, that time change would have brought a veil over the eyes and souls of Adam and Eve as they were thrust out of God's presence. Time became the veil, because we do not have the ability to be in two different reference time frames at the same moment.

GOD'S WORD

God taught Joseph Smith, "For *the word of the Lord is truth*, and whatsoever is *truth is light*, and whatsoever is *light is Spirit*, even *the Spirit of Jesus Christ*."[29] When Moses saw the magnitude of the creations of God, he asked God how he created the world.[30] God answered, "And *by the word of my power, have I created them, which is mine Only Begotten Son*, who is full of grace and truth. And worlds without number have I created; and I also created them for mine own purpose; and by the Son I created them, which is mine Only Begotten. . . . and there is no end to my works, neither to my words."[31]

God created the universe by the word of his power, and he has given that power to Christ. It is not just poetic that John begins his testimony of Christ by calling him "the Word." It is also a declaration of Christ's spiritual and physical power. "In the beginning was the Word, and the Word was with God, and the Word was God. The same was in the beginning with God. All things were made by him; and without him was not any thing made that was made. In him was life; and the life was the light of men. And the light shineth in darkness; and the darkness comprehended it not."[32] It was the very power of spoken words which organized worlds and organized us. "[B]y mine Only Begotten I created these things; yea, in the beginning I created the heaven, and the earth upon which thou standeth. . . . and *this I did by the word of my power, and it was done as I spake*."[33]

Some Hebrew scholars think that words contain the mysteries of God. They think that words not only have power, but the very letters themselves have meaning. To know the name of God is to know God and his secrets. To these scholars, the words themselves contain the power to "Let there be light." Although we do not understand how mere words have power, we all have been moved by such words as, "I love you," or "I know that Christ atoned for my personal sins and I am so grateful for his love." We can fill a room with the light of love, the spirit of Christ, because the words we speak can create light in others. We know that by the spirit, a testimony can create the new light of a testimony in someone else. "My *voice* is Spirit; my Spirit is truth; truth abideth and hath no end; and if it be in you it shall abound."[34]

Christ testified of his own creative powers, declaring, "I am Jesus Christ the Son of God. I created the heavens and the earth, and all things that in them are. I was with the Father from the beginning."[35] Paul wrote that by Christ "were all things created, that are in heaven, and that are in earth, visible and invisible, whether they be thrones, or dominions, or principalities, or powers: all things were created by him, and for him; And he is before all things, and by him all things consist."[36] From Abraham to the present day, prophets have declared the place of Christ, the creator God, in preparing worlds for our progression. King Benjamin's words are as inspiring as any: "The Lord Omnipotent who reigneth, who was, and is from all eternity to all eternity, shall come down from heaven among the children of men, . . . And he shall be called Jesus Christ, the Son of God, the Father of heaven and earth, the Creator of all things from the beginning."[37]

God spoke, and by the power of his word, matter obeyed.[38] God spoke, and light was organized. God spoke, and matter was ordered into elements. God spoke, and worlds were created out of chaos. That God was Jesus Christ. He had obtained enough light in the pre-mortal world to have elements obey the power of his words, moving matter into energy and energy into matter, creating the earth and all the celestial bodies in the heavens.[39]

In one of the most profound visions received by man, Christ is revealed as the creator and the power of the sun, moon, earth and stars. Christ's light is what maintains all light and power throughout the universe, "which light proceedeth forth from the presence of God to fill the immensity of space —The light which is in all things, which giveth life to all things, which is the law by which all things are governed, even the power of God who sitteth upon his throne, who is in the bosom of eternity, who is in the midst of all things."[40]

The Light of Christ is also the governing law of the universe which controls how heavenly bodies relate to each other. Christ taught Joseph Smith that there is a law for each and every kingdom, and God "hath given a law unto all things, by which *they move in their times and their seasons....* And their courses are fixed, even the courses of the heavens and the earth, which comprehend the earth and all the planets. And *they give light to each other in their times and in their seasons,* in their minutes, in their hours, in their days, in their weeks, in their months, in their years—all these are one year with God, but not with man. *The earth rolls upon her wings, and the sun giveth his light by day, and the moon giveth her light by night, and the stars also give their light, as they roll upon their wings in their glory, in the midst of the power of God.*"[41]

Besides the beauty of its poetic verse, this revelation brings up a visual picture of the grandeur of not only the light of Christ, but of the two parts of reality. The earth and stars in their orbits roll upon their wings in heaven where all heavenly bodies share their light of Christ with each other and give light to the earth and all the planets. It is a visual picture not only of the omnipotence and omnipresence of God, but of the universal interconnectedness of all things in the heavens. It is a dramatic picture expressing both faces of the universe, the individual physical bodies of light and the spiritual togetherness of all things throughout the cosmos with Christ in and through all and the power thereof.

Chapter 9
Jesus Christ: God of Light Comes to Earth

"I am the light of the world" (John 8:12)

CHRIST CONDESCENDS TO GIVE UP HIS LIGHT

With his birth into mortality, Christ began his final journey to atone for our sins. With his birth Christ gave up a portion of his Father's glory which he had already accumulated in the pre-mortal existence. "And now, O Father, glorify thou me with thine own self with the glory which I had with thee before the world was."[1] The ultimate loss of light and glory came to Jesus in Gethsemane and ended on the cross. But the birth of Christ in the flesh was the first step in the condescension of God. After seeing the virgin Mary, Nephi was asked by an angel, "Knowest thou the condescension of God?" Nephi didn't know, but answered, "I know that he loveth his children; nevertheless, I do not know the meaning of all things." The angel then answered his own question. "Behold the virgin whom thou seest is the mother of the Son of God, after the manner of the flesh." The virgin was then carried away by the spirit and when she returned, Nephi looked and beheld "the virgin again, bearing a child in her arms. And the angel said . . . Behold the Lamb of God, yea, even the Son of the Eternal Father!"[2]

The God Christ, having assimilated in pre-mortal life all the light and glory of his Father, agreed to give up a portion of that light to be born into mortality.[3] Christ's Father, having already shared his glory and light with his firstborn in the spirit, agreed to endow the mortal Christ with his genes. Being a god in mortality, Christ could then assimilate light and power in the flesh by descending below all things.[4] Christ became God the Creator by inheritance, being the firstborn in the spirit, but he became God the Savior by being the only begotten of the Father in the flesh.[5] Mary, a mortal, was his mother, and God the eternal Father, was his Father.[6] Elder Bruce R. McConkie wrote, "This then is the condescension of God [the Father]—that a God should beget a man; that an Immortal Parent should father a mortal Son; that [Jesus Christ,] the Creator of all things from the beginning should step down from his high state of exaltation and be, for a moment, like one of the creatures of his creating."[7]

CHRIST ON EARTH: I AM LIGHT, I AM GOD, COME FOLLOW ME

The gospel according to JOHN is one of the most important books ever written, not only because it was written by the apostle whom Christ loved, but it is a first-hand testimony of the divinity of our Savior. Christ taught Joseph Smith that after John saw Christ's glory in the beginning, before the world was, John wrote, "Therefore, in the beginning the Word was, for he was the Word, even the messenger of salvation—*The light and the Redeemer of the world;* the Spirit of truth, who came into the world, because the world was made by him, and *in him was the life of men and the light of men.* The worlds were made by him; men were made by him; all things were made by him, and through him, and of him. *And I, John, bear record that I beheld his glory, as the glory of the Only Begotten of the Father, full of grace and truth, even the Spirit of truth, which came and dwelt in the flesh, and dwelt among us.*"[8]

John teaches us that the God who created all things, including the organization of physical light, is himself all the variables of both physical and spiritual light—grace, truth and life. Christ's life on earth was a declaration of his own divinity, his light, his power and his glory, not only in the way he lived and died, but in his personal proclamation to the world that he was the Savior. To the Samaritan woman who gave him drink, Christ promised everlasting, living water. The woman didn't understand Christ's statement, but answered, "I know that Messias cometh, which is called Christ: when he is come, he will tell us all things. Jesus saith unto her, *I that speak unto thee am he.*"[9]

To the Jews, Christ declared, "If God were your Father, ye would love me: for I proceedeth forth and came from God; neither came I of myself but he sent me. . . . Your father Abraham rejoiced to see my day: and he saw it, and was glad. Then said the Jews unto him, Thou are not yet fifty years old, and hast thou seen Abraham? Jesus said unto them, Verily, verily, I say unto you, *Before Abraham was, I am.*"[10] The Jews then picked up stones to kill Christ because the message was clear. Christ revealed that he was the great I Am, the Jehovah of the Old Testament, the very God Creator. The light of Christ was too much and their darkness was too deep to accept the truth of Christ's declaration.

The unbelieving Jews returned, telling Christ to stop making them doubt. If he were the Christ, tell them. Christ reminded them he had just told them, but they didn't believe him. He then answered their questions again, "*I and my Father are one.*" Whereupon the Jews again picked up stones to kill him. Christ said he had performed many good works, and asked for which good work he was to be stoned. The Jews responded that it was not for good works, "but for blasphemy; and because that thou, being a man, makest thyself God. Jesus answered them, Is it not written in your law, I said, Ye are gods? If he called them gods, unto whom the word of God came, and the scripture cannot be broken; Say ye of him, whom the Father hath sanctified, and sent into the world, Thou blasphemest; because I said, *I am the Son of God?*"[11] The Jews had no doubt about what Christ was saying, for they sought again to take his life. They just did not believe Christ's declaration of his divinity.

Christ testified not only that he was the Son of God but that only through him can we be resurrected and receive eternal life. Christ taught that "no man hath seen God at any time, except he hath borne record of the Son; for except it is through him no man can be saved."[12] He declared himself "the light of the world, . . . the light of life,"[13] "the way, the truth, and the life: no man cometh unto the Father, but by me."[14] He revealed himself as "the living bread which came down from heaven: if any man eat of this bread, he shall live for ever: and the bread that I will give is my flesh, which I will give for the life of the world."[15] Christ said, "I am the resurrection, and the life: he that believeth in me, though he were dead, yet shall he live."[16]

Here is Christ's call to the world, "I am God! Follow me." It is as sure and powerful as his being. It is as clear as is his light. It is as reassuring and peaceful as is his love. It is as unmistakable and piercing as the burning of his spirit within us. Christ leaves no doubt about his role in coming to earth. It was to glorify his Father. It was to expiate for our physical and spiritual lives. It was to atone for the lost light we all suffer because of our sins. B. H. Roberts wrote that "Jesus came 'to save' by restoring the spiritual and the physical life of man. A noble mission indeed, comprising a redemption of the world, the salvation of a race, a task worthy of Deity, whatever the sacrifice might be, and Deity's shame had it not been performed, since Deity alone could achieve such a work."[17]

When Christ gave love, mercy or grace he was giving energy, his light to others. Through the Sermon on the Mount,[18] the Lord's prayer,[19] his parables, and his actions, he guided those who comprehended his light to spiritual maturity. "And I beheld that he went forth ministering unto the people, *in power and great glory*; and the multitudes were gathered together to hear him,"[20] Christ performed miracles for the benefit of those who believed on his words. "The Son of God shall come in his glory; and his glory shall be the glory of the Only Begotten of the Father, full of grace, equity, and truth, full of patience, mercy, and long-suffering, quick to hear the cries of his people and to answer their prayers."[21]

Christ began his ministry on a Sabbath day in Capernaum, where he preached with power, cast out evil spirits, and healed the sick; and because of these miracles, his fame spread throughout the land. The next day he cast out more devils and healed a leper and forgave him of his sins.[22] He continued to hear the cries of his people throughout his ministry, feeding thousands both physically and spiritually.[23] He showed his power over death by bringing his friend Lazarus back to life.[24] All these acts of mercy were but a small portion of the light of Christ when compared to the central purpose of his coming to earth. They were food for the moment when viewed against the full majesty of Christ's power to feed us eternally and raise us from permanent death to immortality. They were sensory symbols to display the grace of Christ, but reflect the deeper meaning of his love which feeds our souls and will lift us back into the presence of our Father's glory.

CHRIST AND THE ATONEMENT

Since Christ did "do nothing of himself, but what he seeth the Father do,"[25] Christ's job on earth was to be about his Father's business,[26] and that business was to glorify his Father by bringing to pass our immortality and eternal lives.[27] Just as he did in the pre-mortal world, Christ performed his mission by obedience. Christ was even obedient and willing to do his Father's will when standing at the threshold of the abyss of hell, fearing the pain of drinking the cup of gall, and praying that it be taken away. When "he shall be led, crucified, and slain, the flesh becoming subject even unto death, the will of the Son being swallowed up in the will of the Father,"[28] Christ "prayed, saying, O Father, if it be possible, let this cup pass from me: nevertheless not as I will, but as thou wilt."[29]

Christ came to be crucified for "the sins of the world, and to sanctify the world, and to cleanse it from all unrighteousness."[30] He was, "prepared before the foundation of the world,"[31] "the Righteous . . . lifted up, and . . . slain from the foundation of the world."[32] Christ's atonement for all of us was the culmination of pre-mortal plans. It was the moment for which the heavens and the earth were prepared. It was the moment on which all our hopes are balanced. It was the moment for which Christ assumed the glory and the power of his Father. It was the moment when the light of our Father was expressed through his son Christ, making whole that which was torn asunder. It was the moment when the full love of the Father was expressed through the full love of the Son. It was the moment when all men's tears turned to joy. It was the moment when the power and glory of the Son overcame all that had been placed before him—the binding of evil. It was the moment when the eternities turned from hope to reality, from faith to knowledge, from sorrow to victory.

Christ brought to the sacrificial cross the full range of his attributes of light which he had earned by obedience. Nothing was hidden or coveted to be held back. From his light and glory, to his mercy and justice, and from his wisdom and truth, to his holiness and love, the entire spectrum of light that was centered in him was set upon the cross to be sacrificed. Jesus, a deity, became endowed with all that could be endowed. He came as a sinless lamb, "holy, harmless, undefiled, separate from sinners,"[33] and "was in all points tempted like as we are, yet without sin."[34] Christ was a sinless, unblemished, almighty, loving God, who presented himself to be given over for an infinite sacrifice. He survived only because of the life that was within him, "for as the Father hath life in himself; so hath he given to the Son to have life in himself."[35]

What occurred in the isolation of Gethsemane and culminated on the cross with Christ's words "it is finished,"[36] was the voluntary releasing of all the light Christ had accumulated, leaving him completely on his own to re-assimilate the light back again. His descent into the darkness of hell gave the innocent Christ the power to carry the lowest of the lowly back up into the light of salvation. Christ placed himself in darkness, not only below the most disobedient of mortals, but below the accumulated darkness of all sins committed throughout the history of time. All light that could be given up was given up. No more light could be withdrawn. The sacrifice was infinite.[37]

It is when we realize the divine attributes of Christ's light, his innocent nature and his willing obedience that we can appreciate the full impact of the atonement. In drinking the cup of gall, Christ gave up all that was native to him, causing him to cry out from its darkness, "My God, my God, why hast thou forsaken me?"[38] Nothing could have been more foreign, or more terrifying,[39] than being isolated from his Father's glory. "I have trodden the wine-press alone, and have brought judgment upon all people; and none were with me."[40] The trial of the atonement for Christ was his isolation from his Father.

Brigham Young taught that because Christ's light, knowledge and glory exceeded all others, *"at the very moment, at the hour when the crisis came for him to offer up his life, the Father withdrew Himself, withdrew His Spirit, and cast a veil over him.* That is what made him sweat blood. If he had the power of God upon him, he would not have sweat blood; but all was withdrawn from him, and a veil cast over him, and he then pled with the Father not to forsake him. "No," says the Father, "you must have your trials, as well as others."[41]

Christ died both a spiritual and physical death, suffering the "pain of all men,"[42] "the pains of every living creature, both men, women, and children, who belong to the family of Adam."[43] Centered in that pain was the pain of birthing us into his family, allowing us to become his sons and daughters. "Yet it pleased the Lord to bruise him; he hath put him to grief; when thou shalt make his soul an offering for sin, *he shall see his seed. . . . He shall see of the travail of his soul, and shall be satisfied.*"[44]

The other side of the travail for Christ, besides that of sacrificing his god light, was that he suffered as a human. He was the Word that was made flesh,[45] and "wherefore in all things it behooved him to be made like unto his brethren, that he might be a merciful and faithful high priest in things pertaining to God, to make reconciliation for the sins of the people. For in that he himself hath suffered being tempted he is able to succour them that are tempted."[46] Like the dual nature of light, the dual nature of Christ as God and as a man gave full advantage for the atonement to take place, wresting the universe from the bondage of evil, and cradling the spent heart from the ills of mortal life. It was not just the immortal Christ who descended below all, but the mortal Christ as well, and in taking the flesh with him through the sorrow of the atonement, he brought back not only himself, but us as well.[47]

CONSEQUENCES OF THE ATONEMENT FOR CHRIST

For Jesus Christ there were six important things accomplished through the atonement. 1) He glorified his Father and asked in return to regain his own previous glory.[48] 2) He suffered the ultimate suffering and gained a greater understanding of obedience. "Though he were a Son, yet learned he obedience by the things which he suffered; And being made perfect, he became the author of eternal salvation unto all them that obey him."⁴⁹ 3) He learned the full measure of mercy in becoming our father. "And he shall go forth, suffering pains and afflictions and temptations of every kind; and this that the word might be fulfilled which saith he will take upon him the pains and the sicknesses of *his people*. And he will take upon him death, that he may loose the bands of death which bind *his people; and he will take upon him their infirmities, that his bowels may be filled with mercy, according to the flesh, that he may know according to the flesh how to succor his people according to their infirmities.*"⁵⁰

4) He gained wisdom to judge, and power to raise others to his glory. "And my Father sent me that I might be lifted up upon the cross; and after that I had been lifted up upon the cross, that I might draw all men unto me, that as I have been lifted up by men even so should men be lifted up by the Father to stand before me, to be judged of their works, whether they be good or whether they be evil."⁵¹ 5) He paid the price, once and for all. There is a finality to his suffering,⁵² allowing his glory to be restored and peace to reign in our hearts. Christ does not have to do it again! 6) By descending below all things he regained full access to the light of his Father, allowing him to be in and through all things and still have a body of flesh and bones. "He that ascended up on high, as also he descended below all things, in that he comprehended all things, that he might be in all and through all things, the light of truth."⁵³ Christ received the fullness of glory and was clothed in light. As a resurrected being he assumed the full range of all aspects of light. "And I John, bear record that I beheld his glory, as the glory of the Only begotten of the Father, full of grace and

truth, even the Spirit of truth, . . . that he received a fulness of the glory of the Father."[54]

CHRIST'S LIGHT IS LAW

Christ told the Nephites, "I am the law, and the light."[55] The laws of justice and mercy are both fully expressed through the atonement, because Christ's light is in and through all things.[56] Christ governs all things through the laws of justice, mercy, and love, justice, mercy and love all being forms of light. To let justice and mercy be unbalanced, one having power over another, would be similar to having access only to radio waves, with restriction on receiving ultra-violet waves. If the law of ultra-violet waves is kept, ultra-violet waves can be used, and if the law of radio waves is kept, radio waves may be received. They are both part of the ubiquitous light throughout the universe. Light is the steady, immutable state of law by which justice is expressed, but it is also the unchanging stature of law by which love and mercy are guaranteed their full expression. God is immutable. His laws are unchanging. In the atonement the full measure of all law is fulfilled. Justice is given its full due, with mercy having its full share, both being maintained by the love of God.

Without the atonement, the law of justice would have demanded that we pay for our sins by the loss of light. We all have experienced the loss of light when we break God's commandments.[57] Justice withholds light from us when we sin, just as light was withheld from Christ during the atonement when he descended below all things. The law of justice was satisfied by having an innocent deity take the place of sinful mortals. The vicarious sacrifice of Christ becomes effective in us only when we accept his sacrifice. Otherwise, the law of justice holds its bond over us.[58] Christ gained the power of mercy and the power to forgive because he had suffered all our sorrows. Through his suffering, Christ moved himself into a position to judge, gaining power to administer all the laws of light. "But God ceaseth not to be God, and mercy claimeth the penitent, and mercy cometh because of the atonement. . . . For behold, justice exerciseth all his demands, and also mercy claimeth all which is her own; and thus, none but the truly penitent are saved."[59]

It was Christ's descent below all things which allowed him to become the law and the judge of all kingdoms.[60] Each of us is an individual kingdom because each of us is an unique individual, with body and soul, and agency to act independent of others. The judgment of our beings is accomplished by how much light each of us comprehends, how much light we accumulate. "For intelligence cleaveth unto intelligence; wisdom receiveth wisdom; truth embraceth truth; virtue loveth virtue; *light cleaveth unto light*; mercy hath compassion on mercy and claimeth her own; justice continueth its course and claimeth its own; *judgment goeth before the face of him who sitteth upon the throne and governeth and executeth all things. He comprehendeth all things, and all things are before him, and all things are round about him; and he is above all things, and in all things, and is through all things, and is round about all things*; and all things are by him, and of him, even God, forever and ever."[61]

Here is a clear picture of Christ's light and power. Christ's power of judgment is present in everything through his light. Christ judges by how much light each of us understands and accepts, which is determined by whether we have kept the laws and conditions of our individual kingdom. Judgment is by light meter! "And unto every kingdom is given a law; and unto every law there are certain bounds also and conditions. All beings who abide not in those conditions are not justified."[62]

CHRIST IS LOVE

"Truth embraceth truth; virtue loveth virtue; light cleaveth unto light; mercy hath compassion on mercy and claimeth her own."[63] Just as the nature of light is to be compatible with its own kind, the nature of mercy is to claim only her own. Truth must cleave to truth, and virtue can be attracted only to virtue. How is it that Christ assumed all the light of his Father? By giving away virtue, truth and mercy. In return Christ received virtue, truth, and mercy, grace for grace, for that is the law of light and love. His obedience to the law brought back to him what he cast upon the waters.[64] "John saw that [Christ] received not of the fulness at first, but *received grace for grace*; And he received not of the fulness at first, but *continued from grace to grace*, until he received a fulness. And thus he was called the Son of God, because he received not of the fulness at the first. . . . And I, John, bear record that he received a fulness of the glory of the Father."[65]

The key to gaining the light and glory of the Father is grace. Grace is the light of love, of compassion, and of charity. We gain grace the same way Christ did, by acting virtuously, by giving charity and compassion to others. It is significant that by giving away grace, Christ not only received grace back, but that he went from a state of grace, to a state of more grace, until he received a fullness. A fullness of what? A fullness of grace. A fullness of love! The fullness of the Father and of Christ is eternal love. "Charity is the pure love of Christ, and it endureth forever."[66]

Love is the basic glue that connects all the components of light. From power to law, from energy to elements, from justice to mercy, it is love that guides the operation of each. In the words of John, the apostle of love, "And we have known and believed the love that God hath to us. God is love; and he that dwelleth in love dwelleth in God, and God in him."[67]

CHRIST AS A GLORIFIED, RESURRECTED BEING OF LIGHT

Joseph Smith and Oliver Cowdery saw the resurrected, glorified Christ and bore testimony of him. "We saw the Lord standing upon the breastwork of the pulpit, before us; and under his feet was a paved work of pure gold in color like amber. *His eyes were as a flame of fire*; the hair of his head was white like the pure snow; *his countenance shone above the brightness of the sun*; and his voice was as the sound of the rushing of great waters, even the voice of Jehovah."[68] On another occasion, Joseph Smith and Sidney Rigdon saw the resurrected Christ and declared, "That he lives! For we saw him, even on the right hand of God; and we heard the voice bearing record that he is the Only Begotten of the Father—That by him, and through him, and of him, the worlds are and were created, and the inhabitants thereof are begotten sons and daughters unto God."[69] Christ as a resurrected, glorified God bore his own witness to his divinity to the Nephites:

> And behold, I am the light and the life of the world; and I have drunk out of that bitter cup which the Father hath given me, and have glorified the Father in taking upon me the sins of the world, in the which I have suffered the will of the Father in all things from the beginning. . . . I am the

God of Israel, and the God of the whole earth, and have been slain for the sins of the world.[70]

The scriptures promise that Christ will come in all his glory to usher in a thousand years of peace. The advent of the Savior's second coming will expose his true nature by removing the veil that has separated his full light from us. The majesty of the advent will surely be both empowering and overpowering. "And to you who are troubled, rest with us, when the Lord Jesus shall be revealed from heaven with his mighty angels."[71] "Clouds and darkness are round about him: righteousness and judgment are the habitation of his throne. . . . His lightnings enlightened the world; the earth saw, and trembled. The hills melted like wax at the presence of the Lord, at the presence of the Lord of the whole earth. The heavens declare his righteousness, *and all the people see his glory.*"[72]

Christ's coming in all his glory is the "day of the Lord" spoken of by Peter.[73] It is the day of transfiguration for the earth.[74] The second coming of the Lord Jesus Christ, is the fulfillment of all God's promises to us. It is when Christ's prayer will be answered. "Thy kingdom come. Thy will be done in earth, as it is in heaven."[75] It is the coming of the kingdom of heaven, to dwell on earth, when "the earth shall tremble and reel to and fro, and the heavens also shall shake,"[76] under the stress of being transfigured to new life and light. It is when the "sign of the Son of Man"[77] shall appear in heaven and all nations shall see him as he is. For "when the Son of man shall come in his glory, and all the holy angels with him, then shall he sit upon the throne of his glory."[78] It is the time when Christ will reveal all his light, from his power of justice to his cradle of mercy, and from his cleansing fire, to his sanctifying light. It is the time we shall see our God-Christ as a glorified being, possessing all power, revealing that he is the reflection of our holy Father, the source of all light.

Part III

CHILDREN OF LIGHT

Chapter 10
Children of Light/ Children of Darkness

"Man was also in the beginning with God" (D&C 93:29)

OUR PRIMAL NATURE

If God is light, what are we? What is our basic nature and what are we made of? Where do we fit in God's plan and how do we take advantage of our position? Christ declared, "I was in the beginning with the Father, and am the Firstborn. . . . *Ye were also in the beginning with the Father; that which is Spirit, even the Spirit of truth.*"[1] What was Christ before he was the firstborn and when was "the beginning"? If we were also in the beginning with the Father, what were we before being born into the pre-mortal world and why are we called the "Spirit of Truth"?

Christ taught that "man was also in the beginning with God. Intelligence, or the light of truth, was not created or made, neither indeed can be."[2] Here is what sounds like another contradiction. Our intelligences are eternal, "not created," yet we were "in the beginning" with Christ. How do we have a beginning if we are eternal? Our primal beings are intelligences, also called the Spirit of Truth because they perceive the light of truth.[3] Since our intelligences are a form of light our essential nature is to comprehend, or to be attracted to, or as the scriptures say to cleave to light. "For intelligence cleaveth unto intelligence . . . truth embraceth truth . . . light cleaveth unto light."[4]

Our eternal intelligences are made of the most basic material of the universe, light, which is the Spirit of Truth. Our innate function is to comprehend other light and cleave to it, increasing our own light and glory. Our inner cores, our conscious minds, our souls, our intelligences, are light-accumulating machines! We have an uncreated part in us that desires to progress eternally. It is by the gospel of light that we are able to progress.

Since our intelligences were "not created or made,"[5] we are co-eternal with God. "Anything created," Joseph Smith said, "cannot be eternal."[6] "The soul [intelligence] is eternal; and had no beginning; it can have no end."[7,8] Since our intelligences are co-eternal with God, we also have eternal characteristics, agency being one of the most important. "All truth is independent in that sphere in which God has placed it, to act for itself, as all intelligence also; otherwise there is no existence. Behold, here is the agency of man."[9] Since agency is so important that intelligence cannot exist without it, any plan suggesting a restriction of agency would be a plan to destroy our eternal nature.

Brigham Young taught "that there is an eternity of life, an eternity of organization, and an eternity of intelligence from the highest to the lowest."[10] All matter has life and intelligence,[11] but, "if there be two spirits, and one shall be more intelligent than the other, yet these two spirits, notwithstanding one is more intelligent than the other, have no beginning; they existed before, they shall have no end, they shall exist after, for they are gnolaum, or eternal."[12] The spirits Brigham Young refers to must be our intelligences for they are the part of us which has no beginning.

According to B. H. Roberts, "Intelligence (mind), or intelligences (minds) thus conceived, are conscious beings. Conscious of self and of the notself; of the 'me' and the 'not me.' . . . Intelligence is capable of reason. . . . Volition—sometimes named soul-freedom, the spirit's freedom, or free agency—is a quality that within certain limitations, attends upon intelligences and may be an inherent quality of intelligence, a necessary attribute of its essence, as much so as is consciousness itself."[13]

Lehi taught that it was inherent agency that makes the difference between things which can act and things which are acted upon.[14] Just as there is a variation of intelligence, there is a variation of agency. The more knowledge and wisdom we gain, the more options we envision. If there is a variation in our intelligences and agency, there is a variation of our light. Each intelligence has to abide "independent in the sphere in which God placed it."[15]

The laws and conditions of our individual kingdoms vary, depending upon the inherent capacity of our original intelligence. We each "abide" the conditions we are able to comprehend. As an individual kingdom, each of us has been given an individual law to abide, depending on our abilities, our light and our agency.[16] What God expects of each of us depends on our innate intelligence, agency and individual development in the pre-mortal life. We are not in competition with each other for the love of God. Since we are not generic bodies and souls, why compare our little individual kingdoms to each other? Surely God understands not only our individual pains, but sees and comprehends our individual talents.

An individual's intelligence or learning in one aspect of knowledge does not necessarily mean an equal amount of understanding in another area of knowledge. We should be careful not to assume that a person with a high intelligence in one area has a high intelligence in all areas. Intelligence may be intellectual, emotional, or spiritual, and these may not necessarily be related to each other. Our ability to comprehend the spirit of God is not necessarily related to our ability to comprehend worldly knowledge. It could also be possible that a person with a bright intelligence in the pre-mortal life may choose to not manifest it while in mortality.

IN THE BEGINNING: BEING ADDED UPON WITH SPIRIT LIGHT

After revealing to Abraham that there are infinite, uncreated intelligences, God showed him that some of the intelligences "were organized before the world was."[17] If our individual intelligences have agency it must have been our choice to be organized into our first estate, to be "added upon"[18] with spiritual glory and light, including love and knowledge. "All the minds and spirits that God ever sent into the world are susceptible of enlargement," Joseph Smith taught that "God himself, finding he was in the midst of spirits and glory, because he was more intelligent, saw proper to institute laws whereby the rest could have a privilege to advance like himself. The relationship we have with God places us in a situation to advance in knowledge. He has power to institute laws to instruct the weaker intelligences, that they may be exalted with Himself, so that they might have one glory upon another, and all that knowledge, power, glory, and intelligence, which is requisite in order to save them in the world of spirits."[19]

The first aspect of light added upon our intelligences "in the beginning" was our spirit bodies made out of eternal spirit matter—organized energy. Our intelligences were clothed with organized light in the form of spirit elements, allowing our intelligences to be fully expressed in a spiritual environment. "There is an eternity of matter," Brigham Young taught, "and it is all acted upon and filled with a portion of divinity. . . . And matter is capacitated to receive intelligence. . . . and . . . matter can be organized and brought forth into intelligence, and to possess more intelligence and to continue to increase in that intelligence."[20] Our intelligences needed to be organized into spirit bodies and then again into physical bodies in order to have access to the full range of light, in order to allow us to be endowed with universal power. Christ was the firstborn "in the beginning,"[21] referring to the birth of his intelligence into the spirit world.[22]

Like Christ, our "beginning" was the moment we chose to have our intelligences "added upon" by being born into the spirit world. It was our first endowment of additional light, allowing us to expand our agency by experiencing light through eternal elements. We were of the same type and generation as Christ, uncreated intelligences in the beginning.[23] We are "the offspring of God"[24] because we each received spiritual genetic material from our spirit parents.[25] Our spirit bodies were conceived by our Heavenly Parents to house our uncreated intelligences. We are gods in embryo, with the full potential to mature and to become like our Celestial Parents.

Just as Christ's spirit body has the shape of his physical body,[26] our spirit bodies have a human form. "That which is spiritual being in the likeness of that which is temporal; and that which is temporal in the likeness of that which is spiritual; the spirit of man in the likeness of his person, as also the spirit of the beast, and every creature which God created."[27] Parley P. Pratt described the makeup of our spiritual bodies as *"organized intelligence . . . made of the elements which we call spirit. . . .* What would we call this individual, organized portion of the spiritual element? *We would call it a spiritual body, an individual intelligence, an agent endowed with life, with a degree of independence, or inherent will, with the powers of motion, of thought, and with the attributes of moral, intellectual, and sympathetic affections and emotions."*[28]

When "the Lord God, created all things . . . spiritually, before they were naturally upon the face of the earth,"[29] we, with our new spiritual bodies, were included in that "first estate." In discussing the nature of intelligences, B. H. Roberts wrote, "There is a begetting of these intelligences, the begetting of spirits, the spirits of men, and finally bringing men forth as resurrected immortal personages of infinite possibilities. At each change increased powers for development are added to intelligences."[30]

IN THE BEGINNING: THE DARKNESS OF PERDITION

There is an antiquity about the gospel of light, and the plan of salvation. Each intelligence who chose to begin progression had to understand the long-term effects of that decision. Those who came to earth accepted Christ as their Savior, and those who will come into his presence in a celestial life are those who again accept him in this life as their Savior. Why should it be any different when we were begotten as spirit bodies into our first estate? Those who are added upon with light, are added upon because they have kept previous covenants, and if they did not keep those covenants their progression was damned from gaining additional light. "And they who keep their first estate shall be added upon; and they who keep not their first estate shall not have glory in the same kingdom with those who keep their first estate."[31]

If Satan "was a liar from the beginning,"[32] what did he lie about? Satan must have lied about keeping his original covenant "in the beginning." The original covenant which not only Satan, but all of us made before we received our spiritual bodies, must have been to accept God's plan with Christ as our Savior. God proclaimed to Moses that he had created "worlds without number. . . . And the first man of all men have I called Adam, which is many."[33] Our world was not God's first organized world, and his plan could not have been concocted after we were already his spirit children.

The gospel is the "everlasting gospel,"[34] not only because its effects are everlasting, but because it has always been in place, from eternity. Christ was "the lamb slain from the foundation of the world."[35] The "blood of the everlasting covenant"[36] has always been in place. It is the "hope of eternal life, which God, who cannot lie, promised before the world began."[37] God promised us Christ as a Savior "in the beginning," when we first chose to have our intelligences added upon with spirit elements. The plan of salvation must have been in place for every intelligence, in every generation of spirit children, from eternity to eternity. The gospel of light is as old as light itself, which is eternal.

Joseph Smith taught, "In the beginning, the head of the Gods called a council of the Gods; and they came together and concocted [prepared] a plan to create the world and people it."[38] The brackets are in the original text and are important in clarifying what was happening in the pre-earth council of Gods. The council of Gods was *preparing* to create worlds and people them. They were *preparing* to put into place the plan which had always been. It couldn't have been that billions of spirits were born into the spirit world and then a plan concocted to give them progress. The plan had to be in effect prior to spiritual life so the innate agency of our intelligences would be respected.

What must have happened in the pre-earth council was Lucifer's challenge to God's original plan and not God deciding for the first time who would be the Savior. Christ was already designated as the Savior from "the beginning." Satan came to the council to challenge the original covenant we all had made before being born into the spirit world, that we would accept Christ as our Savior. "Satan . . . is the same which was from the beginning, and he came before me, saying—Behold, here am I, send me, I will be thy son, and I will redeem all mankind, that one soul shall not be lost, and surely I will do it; wherefore give me thine honor."[39] "The contention in heaven," Joseph Smith explained, "was—Jesus said there would be certain souls that would not be saved; and the devil said he would save them all, and laid his plan before the grand council, who gave their vote in favor of Jesus Christ. So the devil rose up in rebellion against God, and was cast down, with all who put up their heads for him."[40]

After receiving our spirit bodies, we voted again to accept God's eternal plan that Jesus Christ be our Savior, reaffirming our original covenant, which we made before we began our first estate in the spirit world. It is the same covenant we all made before we began our second estate upon the earth. Christ reaffirmed in that council that he, as the chosen sacrifice from the beginning, was still willing to be our Savior. "But, behold, my beloved Son, *which was my Beloved and Chosen from the beginning,* said unto me—*Father, thy will be done*, and the glory be thine forever."[41] When God said, "I will send the first,"[42] he was not choosing between two new plans but reaffirming that Christ would still be our Savior, "Chosen from the beginning."

In preaching another plan, Satan rebelled against God and became perdition. Satan's first act of agency was a lie—an act of darkness. In the beginning when he chose to clothe his intelligence with spirit, he, like us, had to accept God's plan, which included Christ as our Savior. He is perdition because he lied about that first covenant. He used darkness to obtain light. He said "yes", but meant "no", and thus he "was a liar from the beginning."[43] It is the same lie that Satan has continued to preach through others.[44]

Attempting to obtain light through darkness is not a foreign idea. One property of light is to proceed from its source outward. Those who obtain light righteously do so by acting as light, directing energy to others. The darkest objects in the universe are black holes. They exist by forcing light to them. They obtain light through darkness. Gravity acts as the opposite of light by attracting matter and light to itself. When light comes into a gravitational field, the gravity bends the light. Gravity attracts light to it. If the gravity is so strong as in a black hole, light and matter are captured into the hole, never to escape. Black holes are light-destroying machines. They are the ultimate selfishness.

When God created all things and separated them into opposites, gravity was the opposite of electromagnetism, because gravity produces darkness, just as electromagnetism produces light. Perhaps in a physical world of opposites, gravity and electromagnetism, just as darkness and light, death and life, are in balance with each other throughout the universe. Just as the Prince of Peace is the giver of light and life through the force we call electromagnetism, maybe the Prince of Darkness is the taker of light and life through the force we call gravity. That would mean that blacks holes are outer darkness.

Satan was "an angel of God who was in authority in the presence of God, who rebelled against the Only Begotten Son whom the Father loved and who was in the bosom of the Father, was thrust down from the presence of God and the Son, And was called Perdition, for the heavens wept over him—he was Lucifer, a son of the morning."[45] Satan's rebellion brought war in heaven,[46] and thus, "Satan as lightning [fell] from heaven."[47] "Behold, here is the agency of man, and here is the condemnation of man; because *that which was from the beginning is plainly manifest unto them*, and they receive not the light,"[48] With his fall, Satan took one third of our brothers and sisters in the spirit world[49] with him to become children of darkness, none to ever be added upon again with light. Let us continue to weep!

THE BEGINNING: BEING ADDED UPON WITH PHYSICAL LIGHT

When our intelligences, the spirit of truth, decided to pursue their natural desire to be added upon and be born into the spirit family of God, we received our first taste of what additional light would bring us. Our spirit life gave us an increased desire to acquire more light and understanding. Our pre-earth situation gave us access to the glory of the Father, and it gave us a vision of what it would be like to be clothed in additional light. "[God] was a glorious personage with a body of flesh and bones, his spirit and body being inseparably connected, and his spirit shining with brightness beyond the brightness of the sun. We *saw him in his majesty*; and when the plan of salvation was presented to us, it was made known to us that . . . we too, eventually would have the privilege of coming back into his presence with bodies of flesh and bones which would also shine with the brightness of the sun, to share in all the fulness of his kingdom."[50]

Our inner drive to increase in light and glory is an eternal inherent drive in us. It is the same drive that God has to increase his glory. God's desires are the same as ours, for we are all made of light. Our desires to be added upon are similar to God's desire "to bring to pass the immortality and eternal life of man."[51] It is the essence of our beings to seek joy, knowledge, light, understanding, and love. What became clear to us in the spirit world is that to gain a fullness of joy,[52] we had to experience all the variations of light.

In the spirit world we experienced the only form of light possible for our spirits—spirit matter, light as organized energy. The particle forms of matter and light with their additional physical elements were still out of our reach. We could see and feel the light and love of such glorified personages as our Heavenly Parents, but we were restricted from their full power of light because of our infant state. Our physical birth added physical elements onto our spirit elements creating our "second estate." "For man is spirit. *The elements are eternal, and spirit and element, inseparably connected, receive a fulness of joy.* And when separated, man cannot receive a fulness of joy. The elements are the tabernacle of God; yea, man is the tabernacle of God, even temples."[53] Joseph Smith taught that "the physical and spiritual organization of the human being conferred . . . additional powers or benefits on the creature thus organized."[54]

We, like the universe and the world, were first organized spiritually and then physically, each time with additional elements of light. "For by the power of my Spirit created I them; yea, all things both spiritual and temporal - First spiritual, second temporal, which is the beginning of my work; and again first temporal, and secondly spiritual, which is the last of my work."[55] We all have been through "the beginning of [God's] work" spiritually when we were born into our spirit bodies, and again temporally when we born into our physical bodies. "The last of [God's] work," refers to our two births into celestial glory, our temporal birth when we were baptized by water into the family of Christ, and our spiritual birth when we are baptized by fire. We must receive "the last of [God's] work" before we can join our Heavenly Parents as immortal, purified and glorified beings. (See chapter twelve, CHILDREN OF LIGHT: COMING TO THE LIGHT OF CHRIST, and chapter thirteen, CHILDREN OF LIGHT: BECOMING THE LIGHT OF CHRIST) Then God's work comes to an end because we have kept our second estate and become worthy to "have glory added upon (our) heads for ever and ever."[56]

We are "the light of truth,"[57] and we are intelligences.[58] The statement that "The glory of God is intelligence, or in other words, light and truth"[59] cannot be over emphasized. *God wants us!* We are the objects of his desire and his love. We are the focus of all he does. All the preparation for our spirit births; the planning and councils in the pre-mortal world; the spiritual and physical organizing of worlds and universes; the planting of the garden Eastward in Eden; the placing of Adam and Eve in that garden with their subsequent fall; the expulsion of Adam and Eve from their charmed circumstances into a lone and dreary world with all its opposition; the coming of the Son of God in the flesh; His atoning sacrifice and subsequent resurrection—all these events are directed toward us, to let us experience all forms of light. All were designated to help us gain the fullness of our Father's light.

Our inner desire and will to expand is coupled with the inner desire and will of God to help us do just that. Our enlargement is the enlargement of God. Christ is the way, but we are the goods. God works to bring us to his fullness by using light's natural attribute of proceeding outward from its source to fill space. God gave away his light to bring us back to him. He used his light to organize the worlds for us, and it was his love that allowed his perfect son to be given for an atonement. It was Christ's love and willingness to give up all his light through the atonement that opened the path back for us. God's light and glory are expanded when he spills all he has to glorify us.

Chapter 11
Children of Light: Facing Darkness

"There is an opposition in all things" (2 Nephi 2:11)

BEING EXPOSED TO DARKNESS

Our journey with light in our first estate, prior to this earth, was restricted to the spirit form of light. Our intelligences with their new bodies of organized energy were only half "added upon" with light. However, our glorified Heavenly Parents possessed both forms of light—spirit and matter. They were our model of what we could potentially become. Our Heavenly Parents were continually accumulating light by helping us to progress to become like them. As with any loving parent, it was their focused attention on us that allowed them to progress. No wonder we shouted for joy when the foundation of the earth was "fastened."[1] We knew that mortality was our opportunity to become gods of glory and light, like our Heavenly Parents.

What faced us in the spiritual world was the choice to continue our journey to be added upon or go with Lucifer.

However, to continue was to accept risks and the unknown. Our step into mortality required faith in our Heavenly Father and the promise of a Savior. It was very clear to everyone that during our mortal journey there would be failures. Otherwise, why have a Savior? No one was going to make it through their journey of mortality without sacrificing light, not even Christ. Because of his perfection, he would voluntarily sacrifice light. Because of our imperfection, we would involuntarily sacrifice light. God knew, Christ knew, and we knew that we would be exposed to darkness, the opposite of light. Staying in our first estate with our Heavenly Parents prevented us from being exposed to darkness, because God would not tolerate darkness.[2] That is why Satan and his hosts were dismissed from the presence of God.

But in order for us to progress to the status of our Heavenly Parents, we had to go where we could have physical elements added upon us. Mortality was the only place we could gain physical experiences. We had to go where there were opposites, light and darkness, and that was mortality, where light and darkness would balance each other. Lehi taught his sons:

> For it must needs be, that there is an opposition in all things. If not so . . . righteousness could not be brought to pass, neither wickedness, neither holiness, nor misery, neither good nor bad. Wherefore, all things must needs be a compound in one; wherefore, if it should be one body . . . having no life neither death. . . . And if these things are not there is no God. And if there is no God we are not, neither the earth; for there could have been no creation of things, neither to act nor to be acted upon.[3]

"A compound in one" would be like having continuous, uninterrupted musical notes played without rests or spaces in between them. Such music would have "no life," because the silence in between the notes makes the music as much as the notes themselves do. Likewise, darkness helps us see life as it is, as much as light does. That is why Lehi stated that if Adam and Eve had not fallen, they would have remained in a state of innocence, "having no joy, for they knew no misery; doing no good, for they knew no sin."[4]

A state of innocence is a state of not recognizing opposites, as a child would see his or her world. Having "joy" and doing "good" is hearing the full range of music, experiencing life, and choosing, as did our Father, to become the light and not the darkness, to be life and not death. We are faced with similar choices as were our Heavenly Parents: "to act" and "not to be acted upon," to discipline our physical bodies to obey, to be added upon and acquire light and glory. Choice is frightening. Being exposed to darkness and evil, being separated from our Father's light, means we not only accepted the chance to succeed, but the chance to fail. Agency places a serious burden upon us because we experience sharply the responsibility for our own success or failure.

It is not that God allows darkness or evil. Darkness is as eternal as light. God's existence depends on the fact that there are opposites. "And if these things [opposition] are not, there is no God."[5] B. H. Roberts taught that "evil is not a created quality. It has always existed as the background of good. It is as eternal as goodness; it is as eternal as law; it is as eternal as agency or intelligence. . . . The good cannot exist without the antithesis of evil, the foil on which it produces itself and becomes known. The existence of one implies the existence of the other; and conversely, the non-existence of the latter would imply the non-existence of the former."[6]

Since God is not the creator of evil, he is therefore not responsible for the consequences of those who love darkness more than light. God did not create darkness or evil anymore than he created light, law, intelligence, agency, or the elements. All of these are eternal, having no beginning or end.[7] But if he did not create light, how is it, then, that God is light? God is light and law because he learned to love and comprehend them. It is not just that he became compatible with these eternal things. He became them! He actually became what is eternal and that is why his attributes and nature are eternal. He chose to be light and glory, just as he chose to take light from the void in the beginning of creation, leaving darkness to itself.[8]

Beginning as an intelligence, just as we did, God used his inherent agency to obey the eternal nature of light, choosing it instead of darkness, being added upon until his eternal intelligence, with his spirit and flesh, melded with eternal light. He became light and assumed the qualities of eternal light. Since God did not create light or darkness, but became light through his obedience, it follows that Lucifer did not create evil, but became darkness by being disobedient and loving darkness. His being is evil and darkness, just as God's being is goodness and light.

FALL FROM LIGHT

Two adversaries, Lucifer and God, did battle in the pre-mortal world over the honor of God and our agency. They continue to be adversaries, with Satan warring for honor through control over us, by taking our light unto him. The current playing field is the earth, where "opposition in all things" is fully expressed. In our desire to add light upon ourselves, we agreed to give up living directly in the light of our Heavenly Father and to come to an earthly world. We agreed to have our previous light veiled in order to gain even more light in the future. We agreed to have our agency tested and to have our inherent desire for light proven, "to see if [we would] . . . do all things whatsoever the Lord [our] God . . . command[ed]. . . . and they who keep their second estate shall have glory added upon their heads for ever and ever."[9]

The fall of Adam and Eve set the stage for us to take our journey toward added light. It was the first step into our second estate where we would be exposed to opposition, where we would experience life with limited light. Mortality was the very thing we desired and wanted, because it would open our journey to further light. It was the experience our Heavenly Parents wanted for us, because only then could we become as they are. Lucifer wanted it in order to gain access to our bodies and souls. The key elements to make the test valid were agency and opposition.

Those two elements were maintained in the fall of Adam and Eve. "Adam [was] tempted of the devil. . . and it must needs be that the devil should tempt the children of men, or they could not be agents unto themselves; for if they never should have bitter they could not know the sweet—Wherefore, it came to pass that the devil tempted Adam, and he partook of the forbidden fruit and transgressed the commandment, wherein he became subject to the will of the devil, because he yielded unto temptation."[10]

Opposition creates choices and agency allows freedom to choose. One cannot exist without the other. In the Garden, planted Eastward in Eden, opposition was expressed through the tree of life (light), and through the tree of death (darkness). God told Adam and Eve, "be fruitful, and multiply, and replenish the earth."[11] But then God commanded Adam and Eve, saying, "Of every tree of the garden thou mayest freely eat, But of the tree of knowledge of good and evil, thou shalt not eat of it, nevertheless, thou mayest choose for thyself, for it is given unto thee; but, remember that I forbid it, for in the day thou eatest thereof thou shalt surely die."[12] Herein is not only the opportunity of our agency, but the potential sad consequences for its misuse. Adam and Eve were told, "choose for thyself, for it is given unto thee."[13]

God's command not to partake of the tree of knowledge of good and evil can be interpreted as God saying to Adam and Eve, "Here is your chance to take the first step of your journey to a full knowledge of truth. But remember, in your attempt to gain immortality, the eating of the fruit of the tree of knowledge of good and evil is the final step in separating yourself from me and my light. You will die. But, Adam and Eve, you must face spiritual death and physical death to gain eternal life and immortal glory. Because you have agency, you must work out your own salvation, as did your Heavenly Parents. You will be exposed to the depths of darkness and the loss of light so you may understand the heights of glory and the fullness of light." It is a magic moment when we take full responsibility for our agency. It is the moment which opened the door to our choice to come to earth and prove ourselves, not only through our acts of obedience, but through the love and mercy of God and the sacrifice of his Son, Jesus Christ. If Christ was the lamb slain from the foundation of the world,[14] then there was a fall also prepared from the foundation of the world. That makes the fall a significant step in our progression and not an accidental or capricious act.

Even though it was Lucifer using opposites—a lie and a truth—it was Eve who decided to step forward and progress. "And the serpent said unto the woman: Ye shall not surely die [a lie]; For God doth know that in the day ye eat thereof, then your eyes shall be opened, and ye shall be as the gods, knowing good and evil [a truth]."[15] After they had partaken of the tree of knowledge, God proclaimed that Adam and Eve had "become as one of us to know good and evil."[16] That means that they partook of the fruit of the tree as innocent beings and therefore they did not sin, because they did not have knowledge of good and evil until after the fact. It does not mean that they did not break a law. Agency was in place because there was a choice, not because they knew the full consequences of their act. Innocent children have agency to choose, but they are not held accountable for their acts because they lack knowledge in their decision.[17] If there was knowledge it had to have come from Eve, who surely was a heroine.

After Eve was beguiled by Satan, her eyes were opened, and with knowledge, she then explained to the still-innocent Adam the consequences of their situation. It was through Eve's love and knowledge that Adam learned the significance of keeping the first command to be fruitful. It was only after Adam and Eve lost their innocence, by choosing to partake and be added upon, that they realized the full significance, the power and the majesty of their decision. Adam prophesied, "Blessed be the name of God, for because of my transgression my eyes are opened, and in this life I shall have joy, and again in the flesh I shall see God. And Eve his wife, heard all these things and was glad, saying: Were it not for our transgression we never would have had seed, and never should have known good and evil, and the joy of our redemption, and the eternal life which God giveth unto all the obedient."[18]

President Joseph Fielding Smith explained that "it is not always a sin to transgress a law. . . . The chemist in his laboratory takes different elements and combines them, and the result is that something very different results. He has *changed* the law. As an example in point: hydrogen, two parts, and oxygen, one part, passing through an electric spark will combine and form water. Hydrogen will burn, so will oxygen, but water will put out fire. This may be subject to disagreement by the critics who will say it is not transgressing a law. Well, *Adam's transgression was a similar nature, that is, his transgression was in accordance with law.*"[19]

In the case of Adam and Eve, it would be like saying, "If you want to abide the law of the garden of Eden you cannot partake of the fruit of the tree of knowledge of good and evil and stay in the garden. In fact if you do choose to partake of the tree of knowledge, I forbid you to remain in your paradisaical state. By partaking, you will become mortal, death will come upon you and you will then abide the law of the world where you can have posterity." What happened to Adam and Eve is that they chose to abide the laws of mortality. In doing so their act was not evil as we would label a sin, but it was a majestic act of courage, not only for them but for us, because it opened the door for all of us to be as the Gods of light, "knowing good and evil."

One of God's first acts in creating this world was separating light from darkness. Adam and Eve's decision to partake of the fruit of the tree of knowledge of good and evil released upon the earth an equal playing ground for both light and darkness. It gave us an opportunity to use our agency to prove ourselves. It brought us spiritual death, separating us from the light of God. It exposed us to pain, suffering, and to our inevitable physical death. It also opened the way for God to reveal to the universe his ultimate power and mercy through his Son, Jesus Christ.[20]

"And the Lord God said, Behold, the man is become as one of us, to know good and evil: and now, lest he put forth his hand, and take also of the tree of life, and eat, and live for ever: Therefore the Lord God sent him forth from the garden of Eden. . . . So he drove out the man; and he placed at the east of the garden of Eden Cherubims, and a flaming sword which turned every way, to keep the way of the tree of life."[21] Following Adam and Eve, we also were removed from the presence of our God and born into the lone and dreary world, into a hostile land, foreign to our pre-earth home of light, peace, love and connectedness. Our journey upon the earth is a journey to discover how we can return again to the Garden, partake of the fruit of the tree of life and again become sinless, allowing us to return to the original light we had with our Father. That journey is centered in the revelation that through the atonement, Christ is the fruit that hangs upon the tree of life. Christ is the fruit which will brings us wholeness.

CHOOSING BETWEEN LIGHT AND DARKNESS

We do not always see the reality of our physical world, even when the sun's light reveals it to us. Nor do we constantly feel the warmth of our spiritual world through Christ's love, even when it is present all around us. At times we misinterpret because our judgment is distorted, just as many of the Jews misunderstood when they failed to hear Christ's words and failed to feel his light. After being rejected for declaring his God-ship, Christ, in frustration, said to the Jews, "Why do ye not understand my speech? even because ye cannot hear my words."[22] "[Christ] who came unto his own was not comprehended. The light shineth in darkness, and the darkness comprehendeth it not."[23] It's as if the Jews chose to use a radio to see a sunset or binoculars to feel the heat of ultraviolet rays; they missed the magnitude of what was there.

Sometimes we fail to comprehend light because we judge others. Sometimes we miss the light within ourselves because we feel unworthy even after we have repented. We can cover our light with a bushel, denying the power of the light of Christ's atonement to shine through us. We can also fail to gain light if we compare our talents unfavorable with others' talents, deciding our light is insignificant. In the parable of the talents, the servant with one talent feared, judged himself unworthy and hid his talent. Rather than magnify what he had, he lost it all. But the servant with two talents received the same reward as the servant with five.[24]

The other side of judging ourselves unworthy is judging ourselves better than others, which can shower us with self-righteousness and creates the desire to control others. Judging others is the basis of competition in sports, politics, and religion. If I can beat you, I must be a better (stronger, smarter, more intelligent, more righteous) person, and thus more lovable. Self-righteousness is the makeup of religious cults and sporting teams, with their flags, their uniforms, and their songs. They all are saying, "we are different and we are better than others." Our judgment of others is the basis of persecution and the denial of the light of Christ.

"He that saith he is in the light and hateth his brother, is in darkness even until now. . . . If a man say, I love God and hateth his brother, he is a liar: for he that loveth not his brother whom he hath seen, how can he love God whom he hath not seen."[25] God says love him, make no graven images, and love your neighbor. Satan says hate God and your neighbor, and worship graven images which you create because of evil desires. All things are reproved by light, because light reveals the deeds of darkness. "For every one that doeth evil hateth the light, neither cometh to the light, lest his deeds should be reproved."[26]

Having agency means that we are the ones who decide how we will react in any given situation. We are the ones who decide how we will see things, either through prejudice, hate, judgment and greed, or through their opposites, openness, love, humility and selflessness. We choose whether or not to be offended. For "the light of the body is the eye; if, therefore, thine eye be single, thy whole body shall be full of light. But if thine eye be evil, thy whole body shall be full of darkness.

If, therefore, the light that is in thee be darkness, how great is that darkness!"[27] Making our eyes "single" to light is a choice. And making our eyes "single" to darkness is also a choice.

In 1828 there were wicked men who set out to alter the first 116 translated pages of the *Book of Mormon*. God told Joseph Smith, "And their hearts are corrupt, and full of wickedness and abominations; and they love darkness rather than light, because their deeds are evil; *therefore they will not ask of me.*"[28] Speaking of those who do not repent, Christ explained, "For they love darkness rather than light, and their deeds are evil, and *they receive their wages of whom they list to obey.*"[29] Two concepts are revealed here. Evil men "will not ask" God for light, and so "they receive their wages of whom they list to obey." It is a choice to seek darkness by not asking about Christ. We are responsible for choosing darkness if we do not knock at the door of salvation, just as we are responsible for choosing light by eating the fruit of the Tree of Life, the body and blood of Jesus Christ.

We all have received wages of whom we list to obey. Due to our selective filtering, we choose what we see, what we hear and what we feel, intellectually, emotionally and spiritually. For example, we can miss the important message of a movie because we dislike the actors, or miss information in a class because we are thinking about something else. We can attend sacrament meeting and miss the spirit because we didn't bring it with us, or we can pass deprivation with no compassion because we have misjudged another.

We focus on light or darkness according to our desires. We judge that we are right and others are wrong, because that satisfies our desire. Our desires shape the world around us. Because it is a difficult and an on-going task to make our physical bodies obey spiritual law, it seems easier to become a law unto ourselves, which really means not taking responsibility for our own acts, but inventing reality which declares our innocence. We can deny light and not accept responsibility by blaming others for our own situations. We react exactly as Lucifer wants, perceiving ourselves without fault, thinking we are creatures to be acted upon, instead of creatures who act. We choose darkness and rationalize when we feel our situations are not our fault. We believe there is nothing wrong with us when we think, "If you are unhappy, get yourself fixed. You offended me. You insulted me. Your way is wrong and my way is the right way. God loves me and not you. I don't pay tithing because. . . . I don't go to church because. . . . I don't pay fast offering because. . . . I know and you don't. I am right and you are wrong." We can become our own law by blaming others instead of humbly cleaving to the truth and living as if we really are responsible for our own choices.

We sink deeper into darkness when we have chosen to not see or feel for so long that we have become hardened to experiencing any light. In his powerful exhortation to his brothers, Nephi described missing the light as being past feeling Christ's words. "Ye have seen an angel, and he spake unto you; yea, ye have heard his voice from time to time; and he hath spoken unto you in a still small voice, *but ye were past feeling, that ye could not feel his words*; wherefore, he has spoken unto you like unto the voice of thunder, which did cause the earth to shake as if it were to divide asunder."[30] "And that wicked one cometh and taketh away light and truth, through disobedience."[31]

The culmination of a downward spiral into darkness continues when we make our own laws, not recognizing truth, denying all light, and even calling light darkness and darkness light. For "that which is governed by law is also preserved by law and perfected and sanctified by the same. That which breaketh a law . . . but seeketh to become a law unto itself, and willeth to abide in sin, and altogether abideth in sin, cannot be sanctified by law, neither by mercy, justice, nor judgment. Therefore, they must remain filthy still."[32] We can even "call evil good, and good evil, . . . put darkness for light and light for darkness, . . . put bitter for sweet, and sweet for bitter."[33] When we follow our laws, light and truth forsake us,[34] and the veil of unbelief becomes darker over us.[35] Then comes the darkness of priestcraft. "For, behold, *priestcrafts are that men preach and set themselves up for a light unto the world*, that they may get gain and praise of the world; but they seek not the welfare of Zion."[36] Now is a time when good things are shunned as bad, and worldly things are being dressed as good and sold for gain and praise.

Just as light cleaves to light, darkness cleaves to darkness. As we desire light, we gain more light, and as we choose light's opposite we collect Satan's wages—darkness. We choose darkness by pretending that a broken word or covenant is not a lie. We choose darkness when we lose humility. We choose darkness when we trust and exalt ourselves over others and God. Strange as it may be, some look light in the eye and ask it to be something it is not, and then declare that it must abide a law that it cannot. "Behold [Christ] offereth himself a sacrifice for sin, to answer the ends of the law, unto all those who have a broken heart and a contrite spirit; and unto none else can the ends of the law be answered."[37] "Every one that exalteth himself shall be abased; and he that humbleth himself shall be exalted."[38] Light is not directed toward self, but moves away from its source, benefitting others by lighting their way, and in this manner light returns again to glorify the giver.

Chapter 12
Children of Light: Coming to the Light of Christ

"I am the light and life of the world" (3 Nephi 9:18)

THE ATONEMENT: LIGHT OF HOPE

Realizing the full consequences of their fall must have been overwhelming to Adam and to Eve, just as we are overwhelmed when we come out of our own gardens of Eden, having lost our innocence and become accountable. Adam and Eve had their innocence rent from them. They were cast from their position of grace in the presence of God, suffering a spiritual death and giving up light. They stepped into the cruel world of opposites and became vulnerable to pain, sorrow and physical death. They made the final break with their Heavenly Father and stepped into the physical phase of progression. "And now, ye see by this that our first parents were cut off both temporally and spiritually from the presence of the Lord; and thus we see they became subjects to follow after their own will."[1] What we all face, along with Adam and Eve, is the opposition of good and evil, joy and sorrow, pleasure and pain, hope and despair. As we move from innocence to responsibility, we become subject to our own will. Despair may come as we face a world of pain and sorrow, as we begin to understand the magnitude of our circumstances. Despair directs us toward darkness and failure, while the gospel of hope directs us toward light and the promise of success.

The first great hope of light to Adam and Eve came from God with the life-preserving promise "that they should not die as to the temporal death, until I, the Lord, should send forth angels to declare unto them repentance and redemption, through faith on the name of mine Only Begotten Son."[2] In a lone and dreary world, Adam called upon God by following the command that he offer up sacrifice. When an angel asked why he offered sacrifice, Adam admitted he did not know. Adam was then shown the full force of the gospel and the keys of hope and of salvation. The angel taught Adam and Eve the gospel of light and offered hope through the atonement of Christ, "the only name which shall be given under heaven, whereby salvation shall come unto the children of men."[3] That message was so beautiful and powerful "that Adam cried unto the Lord, and he was caught away by the Spirit of the Lord,"[4] and was baptized with water and with the light of spirit.

There is majesty here. Light and the hope of salvation broke the darkness and the despair of destruction. Lehi and later his son Nephi received a similar message of hope when they saw through the "mist of darkness,"[5] "a tree, whose fruit was desirable to make one happy."[6] Nephi identified the tree as the tree of life and the fruit "the love of God."[7] After Nephi had seen in vision the tree of life, he *"also [beheld] a man descending out of heaven, . . . the Son of God.*" Nephi saw "the Son of the everlasting God was judged of the world; and . . . *was lifted up upon the cross and slain for the sins of the world.*"[8]

The sign to Nephi is unmistakable. The tree of life in the Garden of Eden is the cross, and the fruit of the tree is the light of Jesus Christ. Here is the hope of all mankind that we too can partake of the fruit of the tree of life. "Come unto me and ye shall partake of the fruit of the tree of life; yea, ye shall eat and drink of the bread and the water of life freely."[9] Here is the declaration to the world of hope and light, that Christ will make good on his promise to be the light and life of all mankind. He will take our sins upon him,[10] declaring "glad tidings of salvation unto his people."[11] He will redeem us, for "he shall take upon him the transgression of those who believe on his name," giving us eternal life and salvation,[12] for "He has all power to save every man that believeth on his name and bringeth forth fruit meet for repentance."[13]

In Lehi's dream of the tree of life there is contrast between those who believe and those who don't. To Nephi's eye, there was hope in the fruit of the tree, which quickened his understanding, and having chosen to eat of the fruit, his whole body was filled with light, so that he comprehended the significance of Christ's light.[14] Our hope is based on choosing to see the light of Christ and thus becoming enlightened ourselves.[15] On the other hand, there are those who succumb to despair, and choose not to eat the fruit, as did Laman and Lemuel.[16] What is important is to realize that it is our choice to open our eyes and be filled with the light of Christ. If we choose hope, we enlighten our entire beings. If we settle for despair, we darken our souls.

Through hope in Christ we will "receive an inheritance in the place which [God] hast prepared."[17] When we "press forward with steadfastness in Christ, having a perfect brightness of hope, and a love of God and of all men" we move toward eternal life.[18] It is hope, together with her two sisters, faith and charity, which brings us to the full light of Christ. *"What is it that ye shall hope for*? Behold I say unto you that ye shall have hope through *the atonement of Christ and the power of his resurrection,* to be raised unto life eternal. . . . I say unto you that [you] cannot have faith and hope, save [you] shall be meek, and lowly of heart. . . . If a man be meek and lowly in heart, and confess by the power of the Holy Ghost that Jesus is the Christ, he must needs have charity; for if he have not charity he is nothing; wherefore he must needs have charity."[19]

The purpose of our earthly journey is to find the fullness of light through the gospel of light. The important truth to Adam and Eve was that their strength over Lucifer, like ours, comes through hope in the atonement of Christ. Christ's victory over spiritual and physical death has been our victory as well. Casting our lot with Christ is casting our lot with the victor of light over darkness.

There is hope in the infinite nature of the atonement.[20] Because Christ is infinite, his atonement is not an isolated event in time or space.[21] The atonement affects all things that the light of Christ touches, which includes everything in the universe. Because Christ is timeless, the consequences of the atonement are timeless. There will never be an atonement failure, or some place it is not in effect, or someone whom it can not help.

Christ's atonement was in effect before it happened. He was the righteous Lamb, "slain from the foundation of the world."[22] Just after Adam was taught about Christ, God said to him, "Behold I have forgiven thee of thy transgression in the Garden of Eden. Hence came the saying abroad among the people that the Son of God hath atoned for original guilt, wherein the sins of the parents cannot be answered upon the heads of the children, for they are whole from the foundation of the world."[23] Adam was forgiven prior to the physical act of the atonement. Seventy-three years before Christ was born, Alma, "racked even with the pains of a damned soul," accepted Christ, and then spoke as a forgiven man, filled with joy.[24] Enos too, four hundred and twenty-one years before Christ's coming, received the marvelous gift of forgiveness. He was told, "thy sins are forgiven thee, and thou art blessed."[25] Christ's atonement is all-powerful, always present, timeless and all-binding!

THE ATONEMENT: THE LIGHT OF FAITH, REPENTANCE, AND BAPTISM

Hope comes from experiencing the light of Christ, but *faith* moves us to fully embrace the joy of his atonement. Faith empowers us to actually partake of the fruit of the tree of life, which can and endow us with eternal life. Faith is the power that moves our souls to touch once again our God. It is the difference between hoping that a new idea will make a great business, and actually selling the family farm to lay down money to start that business. Faith is putting on the yoke of Christ. It means entering through the gate to be one of the fold no matter what it takes. It is accepting that God really does love us individually.

There is a natural sequence of events that occurs from *hope*, to *faith*, to *repentance*, to *baptism*. *Hope* is the desire to move, but *faith* is the power to actually do so. *Repentance* is choosing to allow the light of Christ to fill our being and cleanse us. Empty is the absence of something. When a container is filled, emptiness is gone, because there is something in the container. We don't dwell on our past empty portion. We are the container, the vessel, the receiver of light. If we are empty of light, darkness is in us. Light and darkness cannot be present together, any more than fullness and emptiness can be present in the same place. Evil and darkness are the absence of good and light. Darkness cannot comprehend light or cleave to it any more than emptiness can be present in a full vessel. We cannot fill our vessels with light by concentrating on removing darkness, anymore than we can fill a container by concentrating on its emptiness. We only fill our vessels by bringing light into us to replace the darkness.

Faith and repentance open up our souls and let the light of Christ pour in. They let us accept the atonement, by hanging our vessels on the cross with Christ, so we can be filled with his love. "And I will fasten him as a nail in a sure place; and he shall be for a glorious throne to his father's house. And they shall hang upon him all the glory of his father's house, the offspring and the issue, all vessels of small quantity, from the vessels of cups, even to all the vessels of flagons"[26] It is not our darkness and sins which differentiate us. We "all have sinned"[27] and will continue to sin and fall short throughout mortality. It is how we fill our empty vessels with light through hope, faith, and repentance, which distinguish Christ's disciples from the rest of the world.

Faith empowers us to move toward the light, but repentance is the actual work that changes our direction. Repentance is what pivots us from a position of not seeing light and opens us to the light. It is the energy we produce to bring our sacrifice to Christ. That sacrifice is the sacrifice of giving up our sins and the first fruit we produce in releasing the darkness in us. Repentance is not the only work we will do, but the first work we do, to bring forth fruit. "[Christ] has all power to save every man that believeth on his name [i.e., has faith] and bringeth forth fruit meet for repentance" [i.e., does the work].[28]

Faith gives us the power, *repentance* is the work, and *baptism* is our signature on the contract. But baptism is more than just placing our name upon a piece of paper. Being immersed in water is signing the contract with our entire being, by becoming born again, through the light of Christ. Our baptismal contract is very simple and yet very difficult: we promise *always* to remember him, so we will *always* remember to be obedient, and he promises to *give us light*.[29] Christ promises to be merciful, and to cradle us with the warmth of his light, to help us continue to remember him.

Our baptism is our new birth into the family of Christ. His labor of the atonement birthed us to become his sons and his daughters.[30] Christ gave us *physical life*, because his light is the life force throughout the universe.[31] When we are baptized, Christ gives us *spiritual life* through the grace of his atonement.[32] We become a part of Christ and are born anew by new light coming into us. He is in us. We are in him.[33] We are connected to him through sharing the energy of his spiritual light. When we come into the family of Christ, our light extends even further and fuses with the light of Christ, and we become one with him, his children.

After we are baptized, Stephen Robinson wrote that "even though we are still personally imperfect, we are declared to be innocent because *he* is innocent and we are *part* of Him. . . . We are incorporated into Christ and receive a new joint identity; we are no longer just ourselves—we are now Christ and he is us. Once these steps have been taken, [faith, repentance, and baptism] we become part of Christ. . . . and we are justified through the grace of Christ our Savior. In other words,. . . His righteousness is therefore ours too. . . . Since we are one with Christ, we receive credit for what Christ has done, and it is his infinite merit rather than our own flawed performances that finally secures a "not guilty" verdict for the new creatures we become in and with Christ."[34]

Being declared innocent because Christ is innocent is called *justification*. In earthly law if we convince a judge we are justified in what we did, we are saying we are innocent. We did not break the law. If we are justified in Christ, it means we have kept the laws of faith, repentance, and baptism. Keeping the law of the gospel makes us innocent because we accept the atonement of Christ. "And unto every kingdom [each of us is a kingdom] is given a law; and unto every law there are certain bounds also and conditions. All beings who abide not in those conditions are not justified."[35] From seeing our first light of hope, to opening our eyes through faith, to producing the energy to repent, to signing a contract with Christ by being baptized, we become obedient to the conditions we are placed under, and therefore we are justified. We then become innocent again, having returned to the tree of life and partaken of its fruit of salvation. "Every spirit of man was innocent in the beginning; and God having redeemed man from the fall, men became again, in their infant state, innocent before God."[36]

Because we all sin and fall short during mortality,[37] by our works alone we are not justified, regardless of what our works have been. It is only through faith, repentance, and baptism, where we use Christ's innocence to be our innocence, that we are justified. "Knowing that a man is not justified by the works of the law, but by the faith of Jesus Christ, even we have believed in Jesus Christ, that we might be justified by the faith of Christ, and not by the works of the law [for] . . . no man is justified by the law in the sight of God, it is evident; for, the just shall live by faith."[38] The law says we have all sinned and therefore may not return to God, because our sinful law-breaking does not justify us to do so. But there is another law of light that does justify us if we accept the mercy or grace of Christ. We become sinless again after being baptized, having been moved by faith to repent, for "we know that justification through the grace of our Lord and Savior Jesus Christ is just and true."[39]

Faith, repentance, and baptism—it just seems too easy to be true, especially for the "big sins" we commit. But Christ said, "Come unto me, *all ye that labour and are heavy laden*, and I will give you rest. Take my yoke upon you, and learn of me; for I am meek and lowly in heart: and ye shall find rest unto your souls. *For my yoke is easy, and my burden is light.*"[40] Christ's yoke is placed upon us at baptism, when we accept him. His yoke is the Christ-like life we declare we will live, giving us the right to say, "In the name of Jesus Christ." When Moses lifted up the fiery serpent and set it on a pole, it represented Christ on the cross. Moses asked the Israelites, who were sick from being bitten by snakes, to look upon the serpent and be healed, and those who did look were healed. Those who thought it too easy to be true did not look and died.[41] Alma said, "do not let us be slothful because of the easiness of the way."[42] It is a choice to open our hearts and see the light of Christ. Christ's light is always present. We need only to open our eyes to see. It is not that we beg God for light and then he turns light on so we can see it. His light has always been available and will always be on. We need only choose to remove the beam from our eye to have vision of what has always been.

Our faith must include the faith that says, what Christ claims he can do, we accept. He really can turn our sins that are scarlet and red like crimson, into wool and white as snow.[43] According to Stephen E. Robinson, the Lord assures us that "it doesn't matter what you did. Whatever it was, no matter how horrible or vile, is not the issue. The issue here is that whatever your sin was or is, I can erase it, I can clean you up and make you innocent, pure, and worthy, and I can to it today; I can do it *now*."[44] What is our worth in the eyes of God? All that it takes to save us—the sacrificing of our God of light!

The light of the atonement is distributed across humanity, going into the depths of all sins, whether great or small. Our varied sins are like the floor of the ocean, with its deep canyons and caves, and its high mountains and valleys. Compared to each other, our dark acts and sins are unequal. But the atonement is like the ocean water that covers the ocean floor, finding every little crevice that exists, filling the emptiness, and covering the mountains, making us all equal at the top.

Our feelings of inadequacy could not be any greater than those of Nephi, who became "perfect in Christ," but still lamented, "O wretched man that I am! Yea, my heart sorroweth because of my flesh; my soul grieveth because of mine iniquities. I am encompassed about because of the temptations and the sins which do so easily beset me. And when I desire to rejoice my heart groaneth because of my sins; nevertheless, I know in whom I have trusted. My God hath been my support."[45] Innocence comes again into us when we repent and allow Christ to hold us and accept us with our new resolve, giving us "peace of conscience,"[46] lifting our guilt, and making us new creatures in Christ. After describing his "pain of a damned soul," Alma remembered his father's teachings about Christ. Alma cried to Christ to hear him. "O Jesus, thou Son of God, have mercy on me, who am in the gall of bitterness, and am encircled about by the everlasting chains of death. And now, behold, when I thought this, I could remember my pains no more; yea, I was harrowed up by the memory of my sins no more. And oh, what joy, and what *marvelous light I did behold*; yea, my soul was filled with joy as exceeding was my pain!"[47]

"What marvelous light I did behold!" The entire message of the gospel of light is positive. It is fullness. It is the easy way, and the yoke is light. It is the only way. It is life, and it is peace, for he is peace and he is mercy.[48] It is just as Christ promised. "Peace I leave with you, my peace I give unto you: not as the world giveth, give I unto you. Let not your heart be troubled, neither let it be afraid. . . . . These things I have spoken unto you, that in me ye might have peace."[49]

ATONEMENT: SUFFERING

Coming into the grace of Christ can bring positive meaning not only to our spiritual pain, but also to our emotional and physical pain. At the sacrament table, as we renew our contract, and eat and drink the fruit of the tree of life, the flesh and the blood of Christ, we do so that we might remember him. If it is eternal life to know God and Jesus Christ, part of that knowledge is to know his suffering, to remember the pain of Christ's atonement, his exposure to darkness. Christ learned "obedience by the things which he suffered; And being made perfect, he became the author of eternal salvation unto all them that obey him."[50] Understanding Christ's suffering should help us become obedient, just as suffering helped Christ become obedient. Besides suffering from spiritual pain, we are exposed to physical pain, illness, accidents, and death, which come upon us for no other reason than we live in a telestial world. "For he maketh his sun to rise on the evil and on the good, and sendeth rain on the just and on the unjust."[51] We live in a world of opposites, in a world which contains the natural evil of physical suffering. We are in our second estate, where there is as much darkness as there is light. If there is any meaning in life, there has to be meaning in our suffering.

Viktor Frankl, who suffered the pains and sorrows of concentration camps, observed that "in the final analysis it becomes clear that the sort of person the prisoner became was the result of an inner decision, and not the result of camp influence alone. Fundamentally, therefore, any man can, even under such circumstances, decide what shall become of him—mentally and spiritually. . . . We who lived in concentration camps can remember the men who walked through the huts comforting others, giving away their last piece of bread. They may have been few in number, but they offer sufficient proof that everything can be taken from a man but one thing: the last of the human freedoms—to choose one's attitude in any given set of circumstances, to choose one's own way."[52]

In gospel words, we choose to open our eyes, and see past the darkness to what light there is. We choose how to use our physical pain and our emotional suffering. Since "suffering is an ineradicable part of life, even as fate and death," Viktor Frankl wrote, "the way in which a man accepts his fate and all the suffering it entails, the way in which he takes up his cross, gives him ample opportunity—even under the most difficult circumstances—to add a deeper meaning to his life. He may remain brave, dignified and unselfish. Or in the bitter fight for self-preservation he may forget his human dignity and become no more than an animal. Here lies the chance for a man either to make use of or forgo the opportunities of attaining the moral values that a difficult situation may afford him, and this decides whether he is worthy of his suffering or not."[53]

It is a choice we make, to find love and hope even in the depths of pain, or to find hate, anger, self-pity and despair. What love there is to be found in pain can be found by having an empathic experience with Christ. How else can we understand our God, unless we use our pain to feel his atoning pain, to understand what love he has for us in the midst of our own suffering and pain? We cast our burden upon the Lord,[54] and have him remove the burden from our shoulders[55] when we use our pain to understand his pain. We become worthy of our suffering when we understand the love of our God, and how he felt. Any pain which comes upon us, whether emotional, physical or spiritual, regardless of the cause, can direct us toward Christ.

Suffering can open us to sympathize with the pains of others and let their energy enter into us. Suffering breaks down our physical barriers which not only block light from moving away from its source, but also restricts the light and energy of others from coming into us. As a result of our suffering, we may feel empathy when other's energy cleaves to our energy. We release our energy through suffering which then allows us to commune with others. It is a variation of the suffering of the atonement—spilling what we have and in return we are filled again by the light of others.

What can be revealed to us in our moments of pain are our own weaknesses, and our inability to overcome on our own. The humility resulting from suffering can open us to know we must depend on a higher power. Power in suffering comes from humbly opening our heart to accept the grace of Christ, through the light of his gospel. "The Lord God showeth us our weakness that we may know that it is by his grace, and his great condescensions unto the children of men, that we have power to do these things."[56] "And if men come unto me I will show unto them their weakness. I give unto men weakness that they may be humble; and my grace is sufficient for all men that humble themselves before me; for if they humble themselves before me, and have faith in me, then will I make weak things become strong unto them."⁵⁷ Christ's grace is sufficient to help us find meaning and even joy in a world of opposition.⁵⁸

Chapter 13
Children of Light: Becoming the Light of Christ

"Ye are the light of the world" (Matthew 5:14)

THE LIGHT OF CHARITY

It is one thing to come into the light of Christ, but an entirely different thing to become the light of Christ. Our return to Christ is similar to the return of the prodigal son to his father. When the prodigal son began his return home, but "was yet a great way off, his father saw him, and had compassion, and ran, and fell on his neck, and kissed him." Like we all have done, "the son said unto him, Father, I have sinned against heaven, and in thy sight, and am no more worthy to be called thy son. But the father said to his servants, Bring forth the best robe, and put it on him; and put a ring on his hand, and shoes on his feet: And bring hither the fatted calf, and kill it; and let us eat, and be merry: For this my son was dead, and is alive again; he was lost, and is found."[1]

Returning to our spiritual roots is not the end of our journey, nor is the welcoming feast of baptism the only thing which happens to us as we come back into the family of Christ. The great prophet Enos tells us that after his sins were forgiven, he "began to feel a desire for the welfare of [his] brethren."[2] When Lehi was forgiven he also had a desire to share his great joy. "I beheld that it was most sweet, above all that I ever before tasted. Yea, and I beheld that the fruit was white, to exceed all the whiteness that I had ever seen. And as I partook of the fruit thereof it filled my soul with exceedingly great joy; wherefore, *I began to be desirous that my family should partake of it also*; for I knew that it was desirable above all other fruit."[3]

A foreign exchange student from Brazil who attended my Sunday school class, and was living with a good family in the ward, became converted and was baptized. When I asked his strongest desire, now that he had been baptized, he said, "to have my family feel the same peace which I feel." Is this not the same longing of our Heavenly Father, who desires that we receive all that he has? In us arises the same drive our Heavenly Father has, to share the light we have received. We feel the basic property of light, the need to move from its source to others. We become reflectors of light by becoming *substations* for Christ's light. Christ's light is like having one giant light source which is intensified by adding mirrors to reflect it, like light hitting a ball of mirrors, turning in the air above a dance floor. We become the mirrors.

After we return to the arms of our Father our journey continues when we pivot and mirror our Father by taking his place, and seeing the next wanderer, "when he [is] yet a great way off," we move toward him, have compassion on him, embrace him, clothe him in the love of the gospel; we put a ring on his finger and marry him to the principles of Christ, and feed him the fatted calf of bread and water at the sacrament table. We become an extension of Christ, by bringing peace and light, though love, to others, and therefore Christ proclaims, "Ye are the light of the world."[4]

When Alma the Older taught the people at the waters of Mormon he asked them if they were "willing to mourn with those that mourn; yea, and comfort those that stand in need of comfort, and to stand as witnesses of God at all times and in all things."[5] They were willing and when they learned they could do it through baptism, "they clapped their hands for joy, and exclaimed: This is the desire of our hearts."[6] King Benjamin put it this way. "For the sake of retaining a remission of your sins from day to day, that ye may walk guiltless before God——I would that ye should impart of your substance to the poor, every man according to that which he hath, such as feeding the hungry, clothing the naked, visiting the sick and administering to their relief, both spiritually and temporally, according to their wants."[7]

Our contract, made at baptism, continues to bring new life to us when we choose to use the light of Christ to see humanity through our new spiritual eyes. Our willingness to give our light to others brings new life to them and their new enlightenment brings more light back to us. "Behold, the Lord requireth the heart and a willing mind."[8] We become willing not to judge the beggar who puts his hand up to us, whether that begging is for money or for love. There is a key in King Benjamin's statement on service. "Ye should impart of your substance to the poor, *every man according to that which he hath.* . . . And see that all these things are *done in wisdom and order;* for *it is not requisite that a man run faster than he has strength.*"⁹ We all do not have the same gifts to give. If we mistakenly conclude that righteousness is related to our innate abilities, to our money, to our power, or to our position, we restrict ourselves, just like the servant who had only one talent and buried it because he was ashamed.¹⁰ He hid his light under a bushel. We produce what we can produce, without running faster than we have strength, and we should not be ashamed of our gift of light, no matter how meager we judge it. The playing field is equalized because what counts is using the talents we have, and not the value we place on the gift.

One of my elderly patients from Poland, having emigrated in her later years, could not speak or understand much English, and was quite poor. Each holiday she would bring into the office a dozen hand-crocheted characters which coordinated with the current holiday—Santa Claus for Christmas, a pumpkin for Halloween, a bunny for Easter, sometimes with a candy attached. They had a safety pin sewn on the back so we could wear them on our shirts. We couldn't verbally converse with her, but we would smile and hug her, acknowledging the intent and the power of her gift. I have an aunt who supported herself on a small salary, but she gave to my poor parents a few dollars each month for years, until all seven boys completed their missions. The gift of the widow's two mites into the church treasury really is equal to the influence of the wealthy with their ability to give thousands.

GRACE: THE LIGHT OF SANCTIFICATION

In coming into the fullness of his Father, Christ "received not of the fulness at first, but received grace for grace; And he received not of the fulness at first, but continued from grace to grace, until he received a fulness . . . of the glory of the Father."[11] Grace is used in two different ways in this scripture, grace as a free gift (grace for grace) and grace as an unearned position of enlightenment (grace to grace). Christ gave light away as a grace, and what came back to him was more light. He then went from one position of grace, of light, to a higher position of grace, until he received a fullness of light. We magnify our light by casting our bread upon the water,[12] or by losing our lives to find them.[13] It is a paradox, for we receive more light by giving the light we have away, and "therefore, I say unto you, you shall receive grace for grace."[14] We keep our vessels full only by emptying them, just as Christ did for us. Our part of the contract is to "remember him," by doing his work, and the work of Christ is giving the light of grace to us.

The best part about giving grace is there is no rule on how, or when, or to whom we deliver our gifts. Christ keeps no comparison chart to record our acts for others. We are not in competition. Everyone can be good enough! What is required is nothing other than a willing heart to give or to receive. In receiving a gift from another we give ourselves to them, and in giving our gift to another we receive them into our hearts. There is no difference between the two. Giving is receiving and receiving is giving, because the spirit is the same. It is a variation of what Christ taught the early saints about those who preach having the spirit and those who listen having the spirit also. "Wherefore, he that preacheth and he that receiveth, understand one another, and both are edified and rejoice together."[15] Whether we preach or whether we listen, if the spirit is there, "both are edified and rejoice together." It is the same as the relationship between giving and receiving.

"For there are many gifts, and to every man is given a gift by the Spirit of God. . . . For all have not every gift given unto them."[16] Some of us give time, and some of us give money. Some of us hold others physically and emotionally, and some of us hold others spiritually. Some of us give by using the talents of our hands, and some of us give by using the talents of our minds. Some of us give prayers, and some of us give fasts. Some of us give up our hurt feelings by forgiving others, and some of us give up our darkness by forgiving ourselves. Some of us give up being victims, and some of us help others from becoming victims. Some of us welcome family members back into our lives, and some of us welcome strangers to be part of our lives. Some of us give up our judgments about others, and some of us give up our sorrows over others. Some of us give to others, and some of us receive from others. Some of us do our works in secret, and some of us do our works in public. Some of us give our lives, and some of us give all that we have, and some of us are willing but never are called upon to give either.

What is important, is that we do not compare our works with the works of others. It does not matter what the grace is. It matters that we are in the attitude of giving, that we bury not our light, but let it "shine before men, that they may see [our] good works, and glorify [our] Father which is in heaven."[17] The grace returning to us will take care of itself. The grace we give is our payment for the grace which Christ gave to us, and we then are doubly rewarded by moving, as he did, from grace to grace.

Coming to the light of Christ is being declared innocent by *justification* through Christ. Sanctification is being made holy by purifying us as if we had never broken the law. We become *sanctified* by the Holy Ghost through the charity of our grace. "They did fast and pray oft, and did wax stronger and stronger in their humility, and firmer and firmer in the faith of Christ, unto the filling their souls with joy and consolation, yea, even to the purifying and the sanctification of their hearts, which sanctification cometh because of their yielding their hearts unto God."[18] By giving, we are made holy, are born again spiritually, and are cleansed through the light of the Holy Ghost. The process for most of us is gradual, moving us from grace to grace, cleansing our souls bit by bit in preparation to come into the fullness of the Father. "The spirit is sure to prevail over the flesh and ultimately succeed in sanctifying the tabernacle for a residence in the presence of God."[19]

Moroni taught that basic to our entire move toward sanctification is that we continue with hope and faith, which drew us to the light of Christ in the first place. "Wherefore, there must be faith; and if there must be faith there must also be hope; and if there must be hope there must also be charity. And except ye have charity ye can in nowise be saved in the kingdom of God; neither can ye be saved in the kingdom of God if ye have not faith; neither can ye if ye have no hope."[20] By clothing ourselves "with the bond of charity, as with a mantle", we bond with "perfectness and peace."[21] When we finally have given all we can, it is still the grace of Christ which balances the scale and sanctifies us as holy.[22]

Our baptism is not just a burial of our sins but more importantly it is our birth into righteousness. We then become knew creatures, spotless before him at the last day.[23] As we deliver our grace to others, we continue to bring our gifts to Christ's sacrament table. The first gift we bring is our broken heart and contrite spirit, but the other gift we bring is our Christlike life. We eat his broken flesh, symbolized by the broken bread, and we drink his blood, symbolized by drinking the water.[24] It is another way we become part of Christ and another way he gives us life and light. His meal is not just symbolic, but brings life, by bringing light into us, moving us from grace to grace.

As we become alive in Christ we find an entirely new emphasis in the scriptures. We don't see the commandments as negative instructions any more, but as positive promises. We move from worrying about breaking commandments, to being excited to live righteous lives and to feel more and more joy. We see that bringing our righteous gifts as sacrifices to the sacrament table is as important as bringing our repentant souls to the sacrament table. We become innocent when baptized by water because we are justified by the spirit and the grace of Christ. We become holy when baptized by fire because we are sanctified by the blood and grace of Christ; we give grace, and grace returns again into us.[25]

DIRECTING LIGHT: PRIESTHOOD, ORDINANCES, AND COVENANTS

Priesthood is the power to direct the blessings of God's glory upon us. This power and authority is the force or energy which comes from God as light, visual and non-visual, particle and wave, physical and spiritual. Priesthood "is the medium or channel through which our Heavenly Father has proposed to communicate light, intelligence, gifts, powers, and spiritual and temporal salvation unto the present generation."[26] Priesthood "is the channel *through which the Almighty commenced revealing His glory* at the beginning of the creation of this earth, and through which He has continued to reveal Himself to the children of men to the present time, and through which He will make known His purposes to the end of time."[27] The Priesthood which was given to Adam was used for the same reason Abraham used it, to seek righteousness, acquire knowledge, receive peace and instruction from God, and to become an heir to the Father.[28]

The priesthood reveals God's attributes of light and power to us through the ordinances when we covenant with him. *Priesthood* is the power, *ordinances* are the physical acts, and *covenants* are the agreements between God and us. Ordinances and covenants help us overcome our separation from our Heavenly Parents by opening paths back to wholeness. They are the instruments we use to bring the light of the atonement into our lives. They are the channels by which light moves with intensified power to connect us with God. "An ordinance is an earthly symbol of a spiritual reality. It is usually also an act of symbolizing a covenant or agreement with the Lord. . . . An ordinance, then, is distinctly an act that connects heaven and earth, the spiritual and the temporal."[29] It is the priesthood which holds "the keys of the mysteries of the kingdom, even the keys of the knowledge of God. But it is through the ordinances that *"the power of godliness is manifest. And without the ordinances thereof, and the authority of the priesthood, the power of godliness is not manifest unto men in the flesh."*[30]

Since the knowledge of God is the knowledge of his attributes and his attributes are all centered in light, the mysteries of God are the mysteries of light. Ordinances and covenants are the keys that unlock the doors to the glory of the Father. They guide the Spirit of God into us, justifying and sanctifying us. They allow us to express our heart's desire, revealing not only to others but to our God, that we intend to come home. Ordinances and covenants bring power into our commitments and open paths previously closed to us. They overcome our separation, not only between us and God, but between us and other human beings. They are the means to express our faith that moves the mountain within us, by allowing us to say, "I will." They let us bond eternally to that which is eternal, because they seal us not only to our families, but to our God and his eternal light. Ordinances and covenants let us show and say to all who see and hear that we will be good and righteous. They allow us to affirm our obedience and mark us as followers of light. They are performed by touch and by words, from baptisms to marriage, and therefore register in the universe our compatibility with light.

Ordinances and covenants create, through the power of our words, a new being, just as God's word created new worlds. Christ said, "the words that I speak unto you, they are spirit, and they are life."[31] Our actions and our words, our songs and our prayers, our benedictions "in the name of Jesus Christ," and our commitments of "yes I will be obedient," all move with power throughout the universe, just like light does, expanding our new beings of light. Ordinances and covenants help reveal our souls to the universe through the power of speech and actions, manifesting that we are new creatures in Christ.

The full significance of covenants is found in the sealing powers of temple ordinances where we are endowed with the power of God and are given rights and access to his light and glory. The temple is a place we can bring our righteous acts so Christ "may seal [us] his, that [we] may be brought to heaven, that [we] may have everlasting salvation and eternal life, through the wisdom, and power, and justice, and mercy of him who created all things, in heaven and in earth, who is God above all."[32] Joseph Smith taught that in the temple the Lord *"could reveal unto His people the ordinances of His house and the glories of His kingdom,* and teach the people the way of salvation; for there are certain ordinances and principles that, when they are taught and practiced must be done in a place built for that purpose."[33]

The prophet Joseph Smith told the saints that the temple was a place to "receive the ordinances, the blessings, and glories [of] God,"[34] "the glories of His kingdom," and the "perfect order."[35] Christ taught that "ye are to be taught from on high. Sanctify yourselves and ye shall be endowed with power."[36] The sealing powers to bind both on earth and in heaven[37] are found in the temple through the fullness of the priesthood. That binding process is the process of our earthly light cleaving unto God's heavenly light,[38] and thus healing separation again to wholeness. "Now the great and grand secret of the whole matter, and the *summum bonum* of the whole subject that is lying before us, consists in obtaining the powers of the Holy Priesthood. For him to whom these keys are given there is no difficulty in obtaining a knowledge of facts in relation to the salvation of the children of men, both as well for the dead as for the living. Herein is glory and honor."[39]

Priesthood functions through knowing how to succor. Performing ordinances and administering covenants are important parts of priesthood function, but *ministering* is the other part. Succoring depends on knowing how to give and how to receive grace, light, and love. "And he will take upon him death, that he may loose the bands of death which bind his people; and he will take upon him their infirmities, that his bowels may be filled with mercy, according to the flesh, that he may know according to the flesh how to succor his people according to their infirmities."[40] Just as Christ's suffering taught him how to succor, our suffering should be used to do the same. It is in weakness that we learn strength to operate light, because it is in weakness we experience humility, feel mercy, and *stop judging*.[41]

The feelings which move us to charity are found in humility and non-judgment. "Cease to find fault one with another. . . . And above all things, clothe yourself with the bond of charity, as with a mantle, which is the bond of perfectness and peace."[42] Humility allows us to be the servant, for "he that is ordained of God and sent forth, the same is appointed to be the greatest, not withstanding he is the least and the servant of all."[43] The power of charity is "love unfeigned, . . . without hypocrisy, [without judgment] and without guile [with mercy] . . . full of charity towards all men."[44] Love is the central power of the light of God.

Our intelligences, uncreated and housed in spirit and flesh, are native to truth. We become like our Heavenly Parents by seeking the light and glory of our God. Truth is light and "becoming" is all about love as expressed through grace. What trust God has in us. He gives us power to act in his behalf! We all are agents for him through being justified and sanctified, through priesthood, ordinances and covenants. In learning and accepting what Christ's atonement teaches us, we declare to him our desire to be good, our desire to have an eye single to his glory, our desire to seek not honor but love, our desire to love and be loved, and our desire to unite once again with him. "Charity is the pure love of Christ."[45]

Chapter 14
Children of Light: Becoming Gods of Light

"Is it not written in your law, I said, Ye are gods?" (John 10:34)

BECOMING PERFECT: THE PROMISE

"Old things are done away, and all things have become new. Therefore I would that ye should be perfect even as I, or your Father who is in heaven is perfect."[1] Christ is not expressing a wish, hoping we could be like him and his Father. It is a command, "Be ye therefore perfect, even as your Father which is in heaven is perfect."[2] What a wonderful promise! Christ, our Savior, will command our old selves to be done away and then he will command that we become new perfect creatures. It is a command by a loving God, telling us he has the ability to make us perfect, and it shows the confidence he has in us that as we understand our true nature we will desire the wholeness of perfection.

Christ's command to be perfect is like the command given to Lazarus when Christ "cried with a loud voice, Lazarus come forth,"[3] and life again came into Lazarus as he obeyed the words of Christ. Lazarus did not have in him the power of life. He with his sisters could only bring their faith to Christ, which then tied them into Christ's power over death. It is like the command given to the leper when "Jesus put forth his hand and touched him, saying, . . . be thou clean. And immediately his leprosy was cleansed."[4] The leper could not cleanse himself. He could only come to Christ and say, "Lord, if thou wilt, thou canst make me clean."[5] The leper's body then responded to the command of Christ, "Be thou clean."

Through our faith and the light of Christ, we are justified and sanctified, and we "suffer with him, that we may be also glorified together . . . heirs of God, and joint-heirs with Christ."[6] Being made perfect means receiving our full inheritance as God's offspring,[7] through a process which moves us from one position of grace to another position of grace until we receive a fullness of light.[8] We can all accept Christ's healing command to be perfect and his promise to bring to fruition all that the Father has planned for us from the beginning. Just as Lazarus and the leper accepted the command to be made whole, we can do the same, "till we all come in the unity of the faith, and of the knowledge of the Son of God, unto a perfect man, unto the measure of the stature of the fulness of Christ."[9]

BECOMING PERFECT: JUDGMENT WITH THE LIGHT OF LOVE

We all will come into the presence of our God and his light to receive our eternal inheritance. Even with our imperfections it can still be a moment of beauty and love. Regardless of their life styles, almost all who have had their lives reviewed during a near-death experience have expressed the embracing love of a heavenly being of light. Kenneth Ring quotes one person's near-death experience: "I also felt and saw of course that everyone was in a state of absolute compassion to everything else. . . . It seemed, too, that love was the major axiom that everyone automatically followed. . . . There was nothing but love . . . it just seemed like the real thing, just to feel this sense of total love in every direction."[10] George Ritchie's near-death experience is a typical description of God's love overriding our imperfect performances as humans:

> Above all, with that same mysterious inner certainty, I knew that this Man loved me. Far more even than power, what emanated from this Presence was unconditional love. An astonishing love. A love beyond my wildest imagining. This love knew every unlovable thing about me—the quarrels with my stepmother, my explosive temper, the sex thoughts I could never control, every mean, selfish thought and action since the day I was born—and accepted and loved me just the same.[11]

The amount of God's love we feel at judgment is not related to how worthy we have been on earth. God's love is unlimited and indiscriminate. He does not love those who choose not to receive a fullness any less than those who desire perfection. He does not base his love on the number of good deeds we perform. He will love us the same if we die today without having done all the good deeds we intend or if we die tomorrow after twenty more good deeds. His light of love is like the sun's rays that fall on the good and the evil. The sun is always shining and it does not block its life-giving heat to those who do not perform righteously. God's love is always there, open to all, shining throughout the universe for all to feel. We just need to open our eyes and our hearts to feel the love of God. The righteous do not have a monopoly on the love of God any more than they have a monopoly on sunlight. Judgment and reward are therefore separate questions from whether God loves us. His love is unconditional!

God's love holds and supports us as we judge ourselves during our life-review after death. We record in our brains every thought and experience we have. We carry with us our own judgment and that is what makes it so potent.[12] Judgment is the time we face our complete selves, for "there is nothing which is secret save it shall be revealed."[13] Orson Pratt taught, "Things that may have been erased from your memory for years will be presented before you with all the vividness as if they had just taken place."[14]

Just like Orson Pratt said, near-death experiences also support the life review after death as being a virtual reality experience where in effect we relive the experiences of life and feel again the emotions we felt then, and the emotions of those we affect. Here are three such experiences. "It was like I knew everything that was stored in my brain. Everything I'd ever known from the beginning of my life I immediately knew about. And also what was kind of scary was that I knew everybody else in the room knew and there was no hiding anything—the good times, the bad times, everything. . . . I had total complete clear knowledge of everything that had ever happened in my life—even little minute things that I had forgotten."[15] "When I say He knew everything about me, this was simply an observable fact. For into that room along with His radiant presence— simultaneously . . . had also entered every episode of my entire life. Everything that had ever happened to me was simply there, in full view, contemporary and current, all seemingly taking place at that moment."[16] "[My life review] was not a review, it was a reliving. For me, it was a total reliving of every thought I had ever thought, every word I had ever spoken, and every deed I had ever done; plus the effect of each thought, word, and deed on everyone and anyone who had ever come within my environment or sphere of influence whether I knew them or not (including the unknown passerby on the street)."[17]

Because our life review comes from memories stored in our brains, we are literally judging ourselves every day. Our judgments about others are really a reflection of judgments about ourselves. We evaluate the light or darkness of ourselves first and then compare that evaluation with our judgments about others. If we see ourselves as loving, open people with good will, struggling to be good, that is also what we will see in others. If we have a beam in our own eyes we not only make an incorrect judgment about our brother, but about ourselves. A harsh judgment of others is really a harsh judgment of ourselves. Unrighteous judgment of others begins with unrighteous judgment of ourselves. "For with what judgment ye shall judge, [including self judgment] ye shall be judged: and with what measure ye mete, it shall be measured unto you again."[18] We "shall obtain mercy" [19]because we are as merciful to ourselves as we are to others.

The amount of individual spiritual power we obtain can only equal the amount of mercy and humility we have within us. Our "confidence [will] wax strong in the presence of God" according to our "charity toward all,"[20] which includes charity towards ourselves. "They [the angels] made it clear to me that we don't have knowledge or right to judge anybody else - - in terms of that person's heart relationship to God. Only God knows what's in a person's heart. Someone whom we think is despicable, God might know as wonderful person. Similarly, someone we think is good, God may see as a hypocrite, with a black heart. Only God knows the truth about every individual."[21]

George Ritchie's near-death experience reveals the importance of learning charity for self and others. "I realized that it was I who was judging the events around us so harshly. It was I who saw them as trivial, self-centered, unimportant. No such condemnation came from the Glory shining round me. He was not blaming or reproaching. He was simply loving me." After feeling Christ's love, Ritchie was asked by Christ, "How much have you loved with your life? Have you loved others as I am loving you?" Ritchie's reaction was to think to himself that he had never before felt love like Christ's. "I hadn't known love like this was possible. Someone should have told me. . . . A fine time to discover what life was all about . . . why hadn't someone told me?" Christ responded, "I did tell you. . . . I told you by the life I lived. I told you by the death I died."[22]

We will be rewarded not just according to our deeds, but also according to the desires of our hearts, and if our intentions are righteous, righteousness is what we reap. God knows our hearts. He will "reveal the secret acts of men, and *the thoughts and intents of their hearts.*"[23] He knows whether we would have accepted the light of the gospel, even if we didn't have the opportunity on earth. We are rewarded according to our will to be good. If we are not asked to perform every courageous act to prove ourselves while in the flesh, he still rewards our righteous desires.

Joseph Smith learned that lesson when he, in vision, saw his older brother Alvin in the Celestial Kingdom. Alvin had died before the restoration of the gospel and Joseph thought his brother lost because he didn't have the opportunity to accept the gospel in the flesh. But God told Joseph, "*All who have died without a knowledge of this gospel, who would have received it if they had been permitted to tarry, shall be heirs of the celestial kingdom.* Also all that shall die henceforth without a knowledge of it, who would have receive it with all their hearts, shall be heirs of that kingdom; *For I, the Lord, will judge all men according to their works, according to the desires of their hearts.*"[24] Alma taught that if the desires of our hearts are good, we will "be restored unto that which is good," we will be "raised to happiness according to [our] desires of happiness, or good according to [our] desires of good."[25]

What is important is seeing that our desire for goodness is what is judged! What is judged is the light within us. Because we all have partaken of the tree of knowledge of good and evil, we all have experienced evil and therefore we become frightened of the judgment. But it is like concentrating only on the "dreadful" in "the coming of the great and dreadful day of the Lord,"[26] instead of seeing that Christ's second coming will be a "great" day for those who have righteous desires. We should concentrate on the joy of coming home into the light of God and the loving embrace of Christ which awaits us. Regardless of what evil we have done in our lives, what we bring to our judgment day is our faith and works, and our desires and repentance that have earned us justification and sanctification. We bring our inner drive to be righteous. We bring the light of our beings.

In the review of their lives, most people who report their near-death experiences, say the two most important questions asked are, "Did you learn to love?" and "What knowledge did you gain?"[27] "He [Jesus Christ] wants me to love everybody. It doesn't matter what religion they profess, what their race or politics are, what their skin color is - - I must love everybody. I must treat everybody as He would. I have to serve as He would. And . . . the other thing that I have to do is gain all the knowledge that I possibly can, and use that knowledge to help others. That's the whole reason we are here, to help others."[28]

The two components of light which we do take with us into the next life—our loving feelings and our knowledge—become the two most important things that God is interested in. God taught Joseph Smith, "whatever principle of intelligence we attain unto in this life, it will rise with us in the resurrection. And if a person gains more knowledge and intelligence in this life through his diligence and obedience than another, he will have so much the advantage in the world to come."[29] The judgment reveals light of love and light of knowledge we have gained while on earth. God "requireth the heart and a willing mind."[30]

We came to earth to learn how to be gods. We learn our role by searching for truths in every area of life, emotional, physical and spiritual. We also learn our role each moment when we feel love for ourselves or for others. Any time new light comes into us as knowledge or love we are drawing closer to our God. Joseph Smith taught, "A man is saved no faster than he gets knowledge."[31]

The love of God is always shining throughout the universe and we tap into it by opening our eyes and our hearts to see and feel what has always been. The light of Christ, which is the light of truth, is in and through all things and the power thereof.[32] Before scientists discovered them, X-rays and gamma rays, hydrogen nuclear-reactions, microwaves, quarks, and DNA, were already there. The spirit of Christ just helped those who were most attuned to discover the "Truth." That truth is not restricted to the physical sciences or to theology, but encompasses all truths, including the knowledge of our minds, of our emotions, of our senses, of our hearts, and of our spirits. Love and knowledge are power, they are salvation, and they are light.[31]

BECOMING PERFECT: BEING COMFORTED

When we obey Christ's law of baptism by water we are justified and we receive the first comforter, the Holy Ghost. As we focus our desires to become like Christ we are baptized in the fire of the Holy Ghost and are sanctified. It is after our justification and sanctification that perfection comes to us when Christ, as the second comforter, embraces us and lifts us into the light of God. Christ promised, "I will pray the Father, and *he shall give you another Comforter, that he may abide with you for ever*; Even the Spirit of truth; whom the world cannot receive, because it seeth him not, neither knoweth him: but ye know him; *for he dwelleth with you, and shall be in you.* I will not leave you comfortless: *I will come to you . . . and he that loveth me shall be loved of my Father, and I will love him, and will manifest myself to him. . . .* If a man love me, he will keep my words: and my Father will love him, and we will come unto him, and make our abode with him."[34]

It is Christ himself who will come and abide with us and dwell in us, to comfort and love us, and he will bring his Father to make his abode with us, and they will give us eternal life, even the glory of the celestial kingdom. We will receive the full light of Christ, and that will make us part of him, and he will also embrace us physically. "Wherefore, I now send upon you another Comforter, even upon you my friends, that it may abide in your hearts, even the Holy Spirit of promise; which other Comforter is the same that I promised unto my disciples, as is recorded in the testimony of John. This comforter is the promise which I give unto you of eternal life, even the glory of the celestial kingdom: Which glory is that of the church of the Firstborn, even of God, the holiest of all, through Jesus Christ his Son."[35] Joseph Smith taught that after we have been tried, justified and sanctified it will be our *"privilege to receive the other Comforter, which the Lord hath promised the Saints. . . . Now what is this other Comforter? It is no more nor less than the Lord Jesus Christ Himself"*; and this is the sum and substance of the whole matter; that when any man obtains this last Comforter, he will have the personage of Jesus Christ to attend him, or appear unto him from time to time, and even He will manifest the Father unto him, and they will take up their abode with him, and the visions of the heavens will be opened unto him, and the Lord will teach him face to face, and he may have a perfect knowledge of the mysteries of the Kingdom of God."[36]

We do not have to wait until the resurrection to receive the second Comforter. Joseph Smith told us it is possible in this life. For example, because the brother of Jared saw Christ he was redeemed and promised that he'd be brought back into the presence of the Lord.[37] There is also a time after we die when we have been judged and not resurrected, that we are promised inheritance in the Celestial Kingdom.[38] "Therefore, sanctify yourselves that your minds become single to God, and the day will come that you shall see him; for he will unveil his face unto you, and it shall be in his own time, and in his own way, and according to his own will."[39]

Joseph Smith explained that those in past ages who had received the second Comforter "saw the mysteries of Godliness; they saw the flood before it came; they saw angels ascending and descending upon a ladder that reached from earth to heaven; they saw the stone cut out of the mountain, which filled the whole earth; they saw the Son of Man come from the regions of bliss and dwell with men on earth; . . . they saw the glory of the Lord when he showed the transfiguration of the earth on the mount; . . . they saw truth spring out of the earth and righteousness look down from heaven in the last days, before the Lord came the second time to gather his elect, . . . and they saw the heaven and the earth flee away to make room for the city of God, when the righteous receive an inheritance in eternity."[40] Eternal life is also our inheritance, and we are promised the same blessings given to the prophets, to see and know for ourselves.

We will see that "great and marvelous are the works of the Lord," just as Joseph Smith and Sidney Ridgon saw. "And the mysteries of his kingdom which he showed unto us, which surpass all understanding in glory and in might and in dominion; Which he commanded us we should not write while we were yet in the Spirit, and are not lawful for man to utter; *Neither is man capable to make them known, for they are only to be seen and understood by the power of the Holy Spirit, which God bestows on those who love him, and purify themselves before him; To whom he grants this privilege of seeing and knowing for themselves.*"[41] Receiving the second Comforter is receiving the promise of eternal life by being sealed with the Holy Spirit of promise. It is the assurance that all which Christ has promised will be fulfilled. It is the acceleration of light and glory coming into our souls, and it is the expansion of our beings filling the immensity of space.

Chapter 15
Wholeness

"That they may be one, even as we are one" (John 17:22)

REUNITING HEAVEN AND EARTH

We are not the only part of the universe that is progressing corruptible to incorruptible. God's dwelling place also has to be as he is, celestial, incorruptible, filled with light, truth and glory. As we must be celestial to dwell with God, so must the elements which dwell with him. Since God is light, there is no darkness where he is, neither in the living beings who surround him or in the inanimate bodies. Therefore, as we move toward celestial life with increased light and glory, the world we live on, which was prepared for us,[1] also must progress toward the same celestial glory. There has to be an eternal unification of the spirit and the physical parts of the universe just as there has to be an eternal unification of our spirits with our bodies.

The earth was created in a paradisiacal state,[2] first spiritually and then physically,[3] and then it fell to its present telestial state, just as we did.[4] The earth is a living sphere, acting according to certain laws.[5] It is moving along a path to celestial glory, parallel to our path, to house those who obtain a similar glory.[6]

Just as darkness must be removed from us so that we can be added upon, the earth, in order to "be renewed and receive its paradisiacal glory,"[7] must have its corruptible elements removed. Like us, the earth must die and be quickened again to a celestial glory. "The earth abideth the law of a celestial kingdom, for it filleth the measure of its creation, and transgresseth not the law—Wherefore, it shall be sanctified; yea, notwithstanding it shall die, it shall be quickened again, and shall abide the power by which it is quickened, and the righteous shall inherit it."[8]

The new paradisiacal life of the earth will occur when Christ comes the second time in power with burning flames to cleanse the earth. "A fire goeth before him. . . . His lightnings enlighteneth the world: the earth saw, and trembled. The hills melted like wax at the presence of the Lord, at the presence of the Lord of the whole earth. The heavens declare his righteousness, and all the people see his glory."[9] "And every corruptible thing, both of man, or of the beasts of the field, or of the fowls of the heavens, or of the fish of the sea, that dwells upon all the face of the earth, shall be consumed. And also . . . [the corruptible] elements shall melt with fervent heat; and all things shall become new, that my knowledge and glory may dwell upon all the earth."[10]

The same light that will sanctify us to abide Christ's glory, will cleanse the earth, and transfigure it back to its paradisiacal glory.[11] In beautiful poetic verse, Enoch wrote that he "looked upon the earth; and he heard a voice from the bowels thereof, saying: Wo, wo is me the mother of men; I am pained, I am weary, because of the wickedness of my children. When shall

I rest, and be cleansed from the filthiness which is gone forth out of me? When will my Creator sanctify me, that I may rest and righteousness for a season abide upon my face? And when Enoch heard the earth mourn, he wept, and cried unto the Lord, saying: O Lord, wilt thou not have compassion upon the earth? . . . wherefore, I ask thee if thou wilt not come again on the earth. . . . And the day shall come that the earth shall rest."[12] When Christ does come he will reveal the secrets of all things including the hidden secrets of the earth.[13]

Joseph Smith said that after the millennium the earth "will be rolled back into the presence of God, and crowned with celestial glory,"[14] where it will become whole, combining both physical and spirit elements, uniting all forms of light, bringing together heaven and earth. Joseph Smith was taught that "angels do not reside on a planet like this earth; But, *they reside in the presence of God, on a globe like a sea of glass and fire, where all things for their glory are manifest, past present and future and are continually before the Lord.* The place where God resides is a great Urim and Thummim."[15] Could any description be more clear of the interconnected phase of light than this description of a Urim and Thummim? The very words mean light and perfection.

Joseph was then taught that "*this earth, in its sanctified and immortal state, will be made like unto a crystal and will be a Urim and Thummim* to the inhabitants who dwell thereon, whereby all things pertaining to an inferior kingdom, or all kingdoms of a lower order, will be manifest to those who dwell on it; and this earth will be Christ's. Then the white stone mentioned in Revelation 2:17, will become a Urim and Thummim to each individual who receives one, whereby things pertaining to a higher order of kingdoms will be made known."[16] How remarkable! The earth will be interconnected like a "sea of glass and fire," like "a crystal" where all things are manifest to those who dwell on it. The earth, like us, will be everywhere and somewhere, having united the two phases of light—energy and matter, wave and particle.

CHRIST COMES IN GLORY

The light and power which Christ brings with him when he comes a second time will lift the earth and its inhabitants to a paradisiacal glory. He will come as the Bridegroom to those who have watched with their spiritual lamps lit, burning from their desire to be with him. Our light will comprehend his and we will be lifted to meet him.[17] "And then they shall look for me, and, behold, I will come; and they shall see me in the clouds of heaven, clothed with power and great glory; with all the holy angels; and he that watches not for me shall be cut off."[18] "For I will reveal myself from heaven with power and great glory, with all the hosts thereof, and dwell in righteousness with men on earth a thousand years, and the wicked will not stand."[19]

We are the resurrected hosts and angels of the Kingdom of God whom Christ will bring with him if we are not living on the earth at the time of his coming in glory. If we are living on earth we are those of the kingdom of earth who will be caught up to meet him. We should "call upon the Lord," with prayer and singing, "that his kingdom may go forth upon the earth, that the inhabitants thereof may receive it, and be prepared for the days to come, in the which the Son of Man shall come down in heaven, clothed in the brightness of his glory, to meet the kingdom of God which is set up on the earth."[20] "We shall see that he is a man like ourselves"[21] and he "shall be in [our] midst, and his glory shall be upon [us], and he will be [our] king and [our] lawgiver."[22]

We will be moved from the separation of the fall to the wholeness of the atonement by receiving the light and mercy which Christ will bring with him, and we will give reverence to his judgment and kneel before him "who sitteth upon the throne."[23] "And he that is righteous, let him be righteous still: and he that is holy, let him be holy still."[24] The glory generated by Christ will be so powerful that our cities will shine from his light having "no need of the sun, neither of the moon, to shine in it: for the glory of God did lighten it, and the Lamb is the light thereof."[25]

RESURRECTION: UNITING ENERGY AND MATTER, SPIRIT AND BODY

The coming of the Lord will be a great day because we will be made whole, our spirits of light reuniting with our new glorified bodies of light. Those who come with him will already be resurrected with celestial bodies and those who are caught up to meet him will be resurrected at that time with celestial bodies.[26] Resurrection is the uniting of the energy light of our spirit with the material light of our body. Our spirits will be clothed with the same type of light that they are already familiar with. If our spirits are celestial, we will receive celestial bodies. In scriptural terms it is called cleaving to light or abiding the law of light. "That which is governed by law is also preserved by law and perfected and sanctified by the same."[27]

We inherit the kingdom which we cleave to, the kingdom whose law we have learned to abide. We are quickened and made perfect and sanctified by the law our souls are tuned into.

"Those "who are of a celestial spirit shall receive the same body which was a natural body; even ye shall receive your bodies, and *your glory shall be that glory by which your bodies are quickened. Ye who are quickened by a portion of the celestial glory shall then receive of the same, even a fulness.*"[28] Our "bodies who are of the celestial kingdom may possess [the celestialized earth] forever and ever; . . . And they who are not sanctified, through the law which I have given unto you, even the law of Christ, must inherit another kingdom, even that of a terrestrial kingdom, or that of a telestial kingdom."[29]

The law of Christ is that we must be justified and sanctified through baptism and grace, and have our souls sealed with his light. We then are resurrected into the Celestial kingdom with Christ's promise that we will be with him "when he shall come in the clouds of heaven to reign on the earth over his people." We then will be *"gods, even the sons of God,"* and all things will be ours, "whether life or death, or things present, or things to come." We will be Christ's and "shall overcome all things" and we *"shall dwell in the presence of God and his Christ forever and ever, . . . just men made perfect through Jesus the mediator of the new covenant, who wrought out this perfect atonement through the shedding of his own blood."* Our bodies will be celestial and our glory will be *"that of the sun, even the glory of God, the highest of all, whose glory the sun of the firmament is written of as being typical."*[30]

There are some who have had near-death experiences who have felt a small portion of God's glory and have understood the connectedness not only between them and God, but between them and everything else. Without the restriction of their physical bodies, it seems that it is easier to feel how Christ is in and through all things. Carol Zaleski wrote, "There is no doubt in my mind that it was God. God was me and I was God. I was God. I was part of the light and I was one with it. I was not separate. I am not saying that I am a supreme being. I was God, as you are, as everyone is."[31] Margot Grey also felt a unity with everything. "I didn't feel apart from them at all; one of the feelings I remember most about them was the feeling of unity, of being totally a part of everything around me and about me. There was no separation at all."[32]

From his remarkable near-death experience, Andrew Petro comprehended being everywhere and somewhere. "I am in the Light. The Light is in me. I can see me in the unending Light. But I am still "Andy." *I'm everywhere and I am here. I can see me as a person and I can see me in the infinite, warm and loving Light. I become the Light.* The light is a form that I have never seen, but it is not new to me, somehow I know it. The light has a voice that I have never heard, but it is not strange to me. . . . The light has all of the answers in the universe . . . and I don't have any questions, because I know everything that the Light knows."[33]

Sometimes the universal light experienced by those who have died and returned is described as love. Just as our beings are already larger than our physical bodies, our beings can expand to engulf the whole of the universe through love. Kenneth Ring wrote, "This magnificent light seemed to be pouring through a brilliant crystal. It seemed to radiate from the very center of the consciousness I was in and to shine out in every direction through the infinite expanses of the universe. I became aware that it was part of all living things and that at the same time all living things were part of it. I knew it was omnipotent, that it represented infinite divine love. It was as if my heart wanted to leap out of my body towards it."[34]

Charles Flynn also wrote of love connecting all things. "Feeling myself enveloped in that love, feeling myself surrounded with the knowledge that came off of it, I felt like I knew the secrets of everything from the very beginning of time to infinity, and I realized that there was no end. I realized that we are but a very small part of something that's gigantic, but as people we interlock into each other's lives like puzzle pieces, and that we are just an infinitely small part of the universe. But we're also very special."[35]

BEING ONE IN FULLNESS

Receiving a fullness is being glorified in Christ as he is glorified in his Father.[36] We cannot receive a fullness of glory unless we are like Christ, unless we are "made equal to him."[37] Christ shall "change our vile body, that it may be fashioned like unto his glorious body, according to the working whereby he is able even to subdue all things unto himself."[38] Wholeness is uniting our spirit bodies with our physical bodies into eternal celestial light. We will receive a fullness when our beings have been sealed by light and we become like those who are light, and we will then look at other Gods and see a reflection of ourselves as we, "with open face beholding as in a glass the glory of the Lord, are changed into the same image from glory to glory, even as by the Spirit of the Lord."[39]

We will assume the attributes of God by becoming eternal light as he is, everywhere and yet individuals, timeless and in time, knowing all and still learning, and one with all and one with self. We will become full-grown adult Gods like our Heavenly Parents, for as God has said, "Ye are gods; and all you are children of the most high."[40] We will become one with eternity by taking the dual sides of reality, spiritual and physical, the two faces of truth, and joining them together as a whole. We will gain the full power of glory, including the power of eternal procreation. "Then shall they be gods, because they have no end; therefore shall they be from everlasting to everlasting, because they continue; then shall they be above all, because all things are subject unto them. Then shall they be gods, because they have all power, and the angels are subject unto them,"[41] "glorified in truth and [knowing] all things."[42]

"And he that receiveth my Father receiveth my Father's kingdom; therefore all that my Father hath shall be given unto him."[43] All that the Father has is his glory, his omnipresence, his omniscience, his omnipotence and his all-loving light, which he will give to us. We will be God, one and the same with God the Eternal Father, "equal in power, and in might, and in dominion. And the glory of the celestial is one, even as the glory of the sun is one."[44] Just as Christ and his Father share their light and are one being, we will share our being of light with the other Gods of eternity. We will become powerful free agents with individual celestial bodies, light in all its forms, with all its power, knowledge and love. Christ's prayer will then be answered, "that they all may be one; as thou Father, art in me, and I in thee, that they also may be one in us . . . And the glory which thou gavest me I have given them; that they may be one, even as we are one: I in them, and thou in me, that they may be made perfect in one."[45]

All God has worked for, all Christ has worked for, and all we have worked for since our first choice as intelligences to be added upon, will come to fruition with the reuniting of our spirits and bodies. Then we will have the fullness of our Father added upon us and we will be the light and glory of the

Celestial kingdom.[46] We will cleave to the light of eternity, and we will be eternal, because we will be light, just as our Heavenly Parents are light. We will be in the presence of our Father and his Son,[47] and they will reveal themselves unto us and we will see them as they are, face to face.[48] We will understand the mysteries of the kingdom from the beginning to the end, and we will see the wonders of eternity, and gain wisdom and enlightenment,[49] and we will comprehend all things,[50] even God.[51] We will be truth and therefore know all things.[52] We will be filled with "the peaceable things of immortal glory,"[53] and with joy, "having peace of conscience."[54]

We will be made perfect in Christ,[55] our bodies filled with light,[56] and we will answer the age-old questions of Isaiah, "Who among us shall dwell with the devouring fire? Who among us shall dwell with everlasting burnings?"[57] We will! We will! We who have given up the darkness and corruption of the world through the atonement of Jesus Christ will dwell with the devouring fire. We who "abide the day of [Christ's] coming"[58] will dwell with everlasting burnings. We who declare with all humility and grace our righteousness that we remember who we are—the sons and daughters of the most high God, brothers and sisters to the light of truth, Jesus Christ. We who desire righteousness will rejoice with our Heavenly Parents in the abundance of life and light and we will understand Christ's declaration of love: "I am come that they might have life, and that they might have it more abundantly."[59]

Part of being perfect is being made "perfect in one" with God and his Son. Christ is in us and "the day shall come when ye shall comprehend even God, being quickened in him and by him. Then shall ye know that ye have seen me, that I am, and that I am the true light that is in you, and that you are in me; otherwise ye could not abound."[60] We will not just be one in purpose or one with God, we are in Christ and we are quickened in God! "And thou art after the order of him who was without beginning of days or end of years, from all eternity to all eternity. *Behold, thou art one in me, a son of God; and thus may all become my sons.*"[61] Because we are of the order of the Gods, our beings, like theirs, will connect with all things throughout the universe.[52]

The key to being whole in Christ is that in bringing us to immortality and in giving us eternal life, Christ, the giver of immortality, increases his own glory as he gives us the glory of the Celestial kingdom. God said we are his work and his glory, and Christ said that as he is in us, and we become one with him, he is glorified through us. "Father, I pray. . . for those whom thou hast given me out of the world, because of their faith, that they may be purified in me, that I may be in them as thou Father, art in me, that we may be one, *that I may be glorified in them.*"[63] We will become the glory of the celestial kingdom and the whole of the universe in Christ and in all other beings with celestial glory. We will be whole with Christ and we therefore will be in the sun, the moon and the stars, and the power thereof.[64] Our beings of light will fill the immensity of space giving life, light, law and power, placing us in the midst of all things.[65] We will be whole with Christ who "comprehendeth all things, and all things are before him, and all things are round about him; and he is above all things, and in all things, and is through all things, and is round about all things; and all things are by him, and of him, even God, forever and ever."[66]

We will not and cannot be separated from the light of Christ, for we will be united with all eternity. In that light, C. S. Lewis' simile becomes more real than poetic: "I believe in Christianity as I believe that the Sun has risen, not only because I see it, but because by it I see everything else."[67] We will see everything else because we will literally become the light of the sun and the light of the Son, taking the place of our Heavenly Parents, assuming the work and the glory of bringing to pass the immortality and eternal lives of other intelligences, and the cycle will begin again. We will then be glorified beings of light, whole, having united heaven and earth, eternity and time, energy and mass, spirit and matter. "And for this cause ye shall have fulness of joy; and ye shall sit down in the kingdom of my Father; yea, your joy shall be full, even as the Father hath given me fulness of joy; and ye shall be even as I am, and I am even as the Father; and the Father and I are one."[68]

Part IV

REFERENCES

APPENDIX A

Light as Wave and Particle—Diagrams

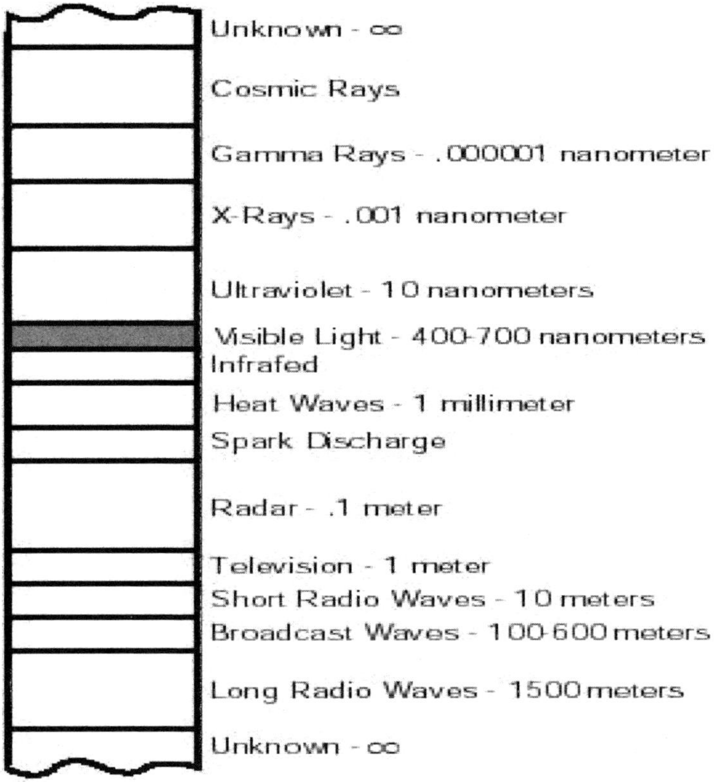

Unknown - ∞

Cosmic Rays

Gamma Rays - .000001 nanometer

X-Rays - .001 nanometer

Ultraviolet - 10 nanometers

Visible Light - 400-700 nanometers

Infrafed

Heat Waves - 1 millimeter

Spark Discharge

Radar - .1 meter

Television - 1 meter

Short Radio Waves - 10 meters

Broadcast Waves - 100-600 meters

Long Radio Waves - 1500 meters

Unknown - ∞

Diagram 1
Reference # 5, Chapter Two
Diagram of electromagnetic light spectrum

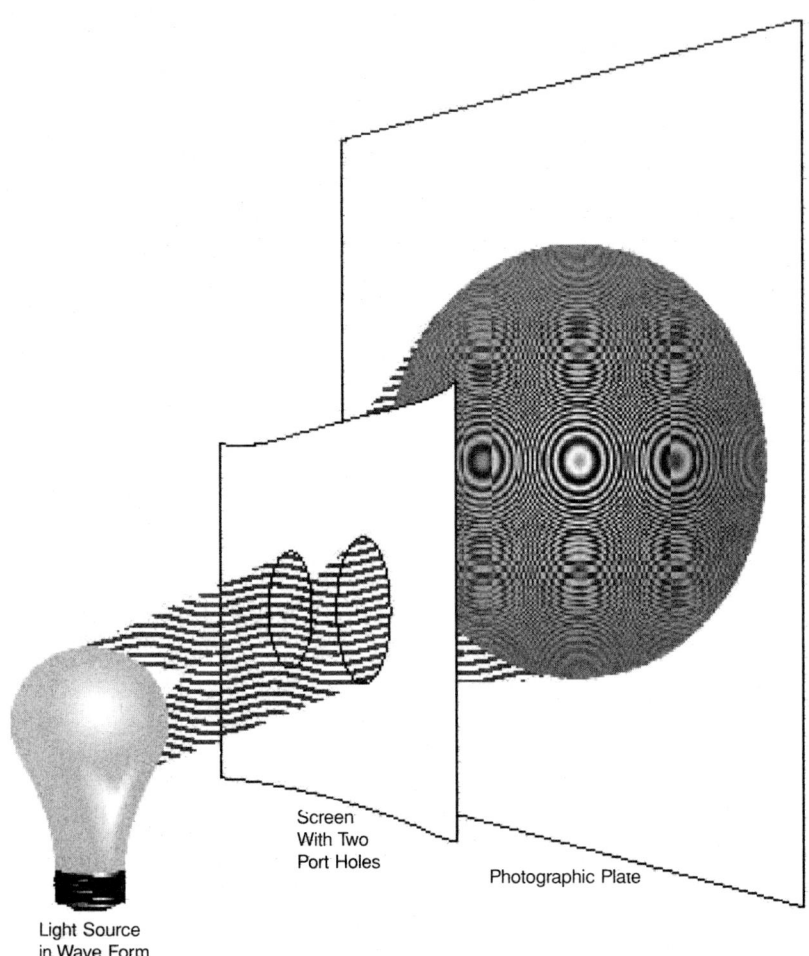

Diagram 2
Reference # 11, Chapter Two
*Diagram of light in its wave form,
showing an interference pattern*

References 191

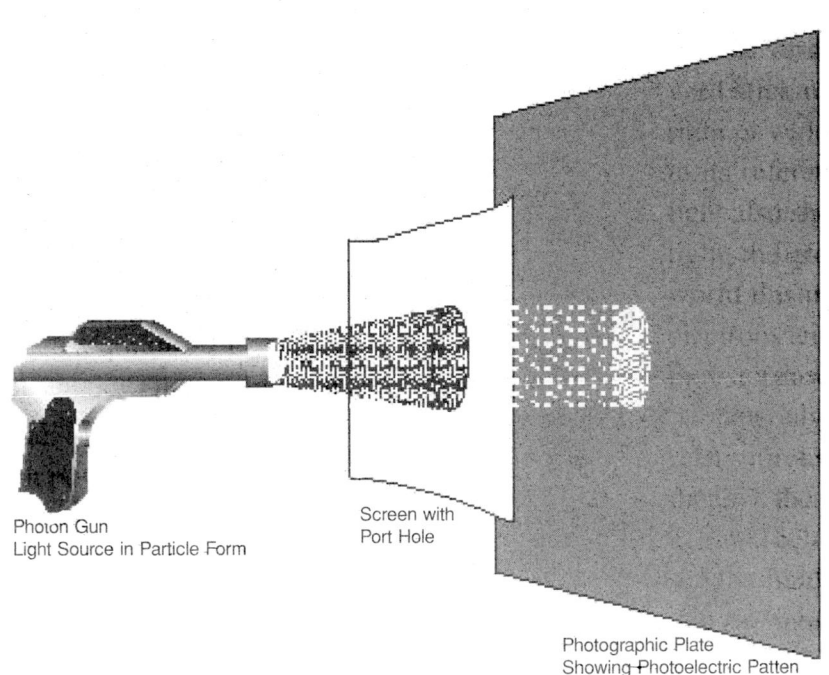

Diagram 3
Reference # 12, Chapter Two
*Diagram of light in its particle form,
showing a photoelectric pattern*

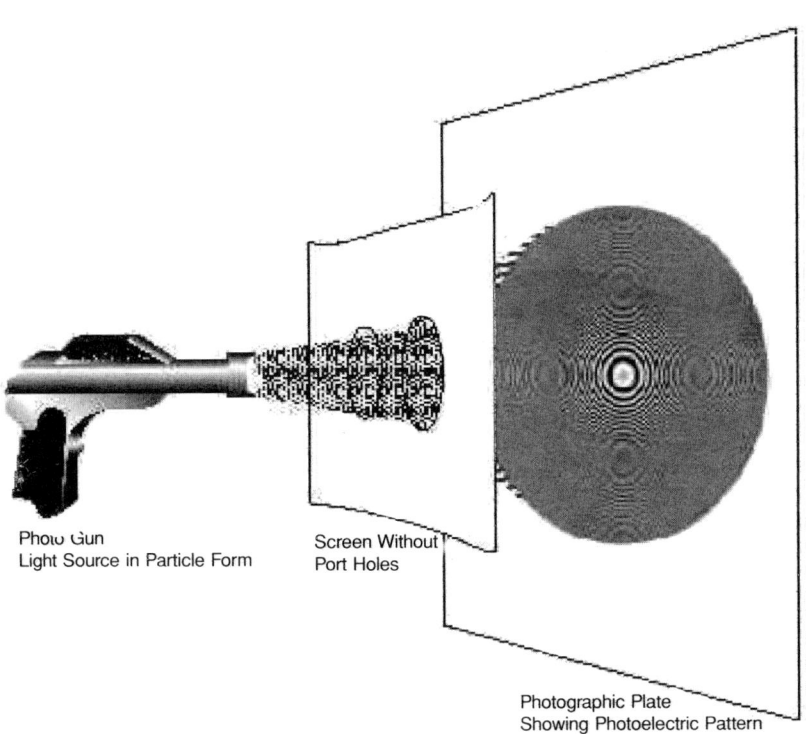

Diagram 4
Reference from Appendix C
*Diagram of interference pattern
produced with a photon gun*

References 193

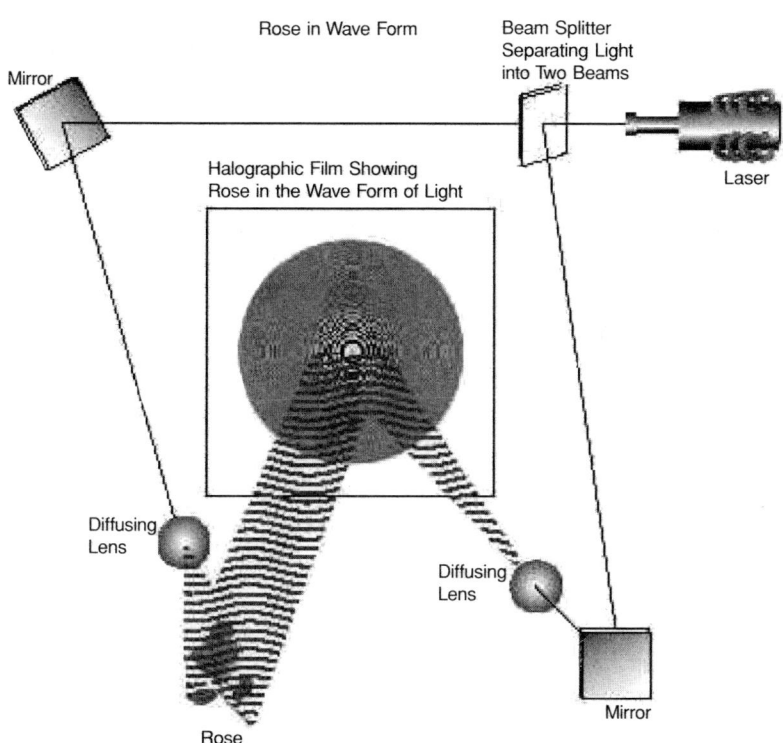

Diagram 5
Reference from Appendix D
Diagram of hologram of rose in the wave form

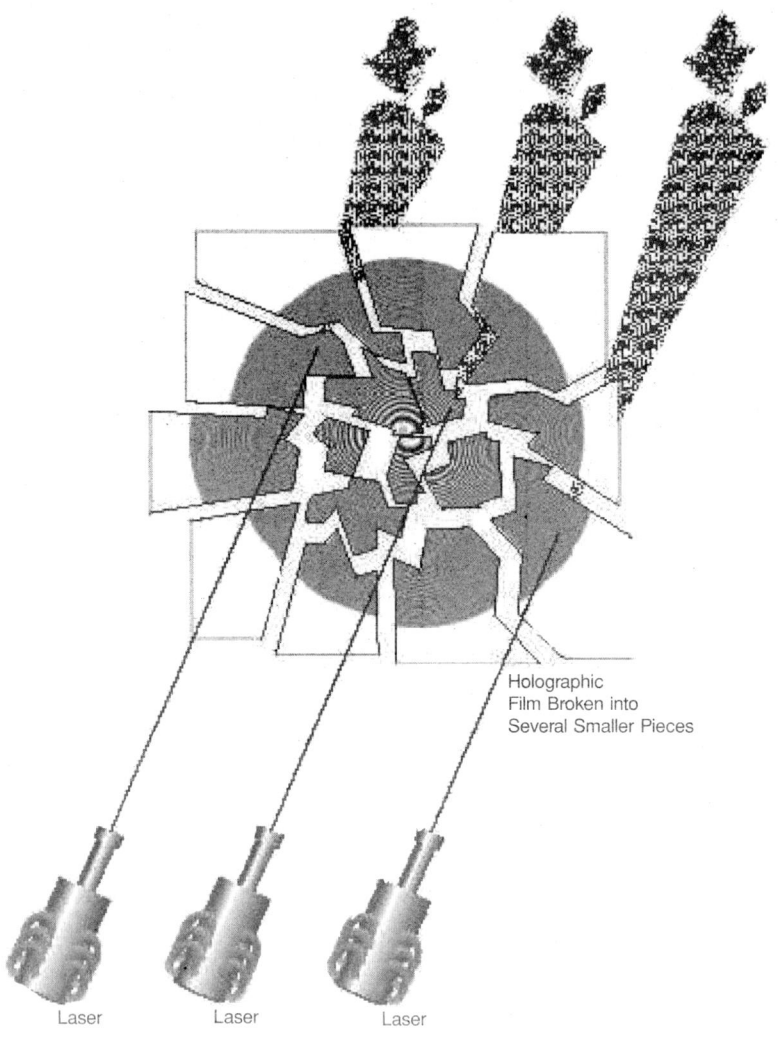

Diagram 6
Reference from Appendix D
*Diagram of hologram of rose
in both the particle and wave form*

APPENDIX B

The Interconnectedness of Light
Reference #1, Chapter Three

Electrons come in pairs which spin in directions opposite from each other. For example, if one electron of the pair spins clockwise the other electron will spin counterclockwise as they orbit together around the nucleus of their atom. If a pair of electrons is removed from the atom and the two electrons are separated and sent away from each other, they still remain connected. If magnets are used to cause a clockwise spin of one of the separating electrons, its paired electron, still traveling away from its partner, will begin to spin counterclockwise instantaneously, no matter how far apart the two electrons have become. The pair of electrons seem to communicate faster than the speed of light and no one knows how they do it.

Electrons will also act as if they are a unified whole. Plasma is a gas with a high density of electrons and atoms. Electrons in a plasma mix don't behave as individual electrons. They begin to behave as if they were part of a connected, larger whole. Some individual electrons in plasma seem to move in a random pattern but a large number of the electrons are able to produce effects that appear to be well organized.

In describing David Bohm's ideas, Michael Talbot wrote, "Like some amoeboid creature, the plasma constantly regenerated itself and enclosed all impurities in a wall in the same way that a biological organism might encase a foreign substance in a cyst. So struck was Bohm by these organic qualities that he later remarked he'd frequently had the impression the electron sea was 'alive.' . . . These were no longer situations involving two particles, each behaving as if it knew what the other was doing, but entire oceans of particles, each behaving as if it knew what untold trillions of other were doing" (Michael Talbot, *The Holographic Universe* [New York: Harper Collins, 1991], p. 38; see also David Bohm, *Wholeness and the Implicate Order* [London: Routlege & Kegan Paul, 1980]).

APPENDIX C

The Unity of Light
Reference # 4, Chapter Three

There is not only an interconnectedness between components of nature, but also between nature and the observer. When experiments are performed to reveal either the wave or particle form of light, what is produced depends on how the experimenter has set up the test. Light only shows us one of its forms at a time and it is the observer who brings into focus which form of light will be presented. To test for the interference wave pattern of light, a screen with two port holes a few inches apart is placed between a light source and a screen. The two port holes act as two rocks being dropped into a placid pool, with each rock producing waves which then interfere with each other as the waves collide. The light shines through the two port holes and shows a wave or interference pattern on the wall (see Diagram #2). Now if one of the port holes is covered, and instead of a lamp, a photon gun is used to shoot individual photons (particles of light) through the single slit, a photoelectric particle effect is seen on the screen (see Diagram #3).

However, if both slits are open, but individual photons are shot at the screen through just one of the opened slits, unbelievably, an interference or wave pattern appears on the screen, just as though the individual photons came through both slits in a wave form (see Diagram #4). Then, if one slit is covered immediately after photons are released from the gun and before they reach the open slits, the pattern goes back to a photoelectric, particle pattern (see Diagram #3).

How do the photons know whether the other slit is open or closed? The particles can't be tricked into showing something that is not being tested for. It is as if the photons know the observer is looking for wave interference and therefore, reveal waves, even though it is photon particles being shot at the screen. It is as if the photons are saying, "Don't try to trick me, Mr. Observer. You asked for wave interference and that is what I gave you." In other words, the experimenter is the one who determines whether the wave or particle form of light is seen. Light responds to the experimenter's test and does not act independent of the scientist. The observer therefore influences the outcome of the experiment.

Electrons obey electron laws until scientists interrupt them and test their wave form or their particle form, or measure their position or speed, or influence one electron's spin to see what its pair will do. When the electron is interrupted, it stops doing whatever it is doing and answers the question the scientists' experiment is asking. The observer is therefore creating the answer. It is like having a thought and someone asks you what you are thinking. By answering, you create a new thought related to the questioner. The new thought is not the original thought because any interaction with someone else creates a new thought. No one will ever be able to listen in on another's thought because by doing so a new thought is created. A person just cannot get inside another's mind.

This same problem in physics was expressed as a simile by Einstein. He described the atom as being like a watch. Physicists can see the effect of the watch's insides. They can see the hands move, hear it tick and see the numbers fluoresce in the dark, but they cannot see the mechanics working inside the watch and they will never see inside the watch. They can only test the effects of the watch mechanics and play with the dials to let the watch tell what it can tell, namely what time it is.

Nature and man are a whole, inseparable, influencing each other, communicating in some unknown way. Nature, therefore, cannot be talked about without including man. Gary Zukav wrote, "The new physics tells us that an observer cannot observe without altering what he sees. Observer and observed are interrelated in a real and fundamental sense. The exact nature of this interrelation is not clear, but there is a growing body of evidence that the distinction between the 'in here' and the 'out there' is illusion." Gary Zukav, *The Dancing Wu Li Masters* [New York: Bantam Books, 1980], p. 92).

APPENDIX D

Holograms and the Nature of Light and God
Reference # 12, Chapter Three

David Bohm's model of the universe attempts to explain the mysterious dual properties of light. Even though his insights into the universe are speculative, they are some of the most exciting of the last fifty years (David Bohm, *Wholeness and the Implicate Order* [London: Routlege & Kegan Paul, 1980]). Amazingly, Bohm's model of the universe is also one possible explanation to our religious questions about the seemingly contradictory characteristics of our Heavenly Father.

Bohm's model is based on holograms, which express both phases of light at the same time. Holograms are produced by using a laser as the light source. Lasers are great at producing the interference pattern of light, because lasers are pure, refined light, usually of one wave length. They are essentially the perfect wave because they don't have a mixture of several different wave lengths as does sunlight. Holograms have two different forms, much like the basic structure of light and all subatomic parts. They have a wave form which is continuous, and a particle form which has boundaries.

The interference wave form is produced when a single laser beam is split into two separate beams, creating two light sources. One beam is reflected off an object—say a rose—onto a photographic film. The second beam is routed around the rose to shine on the same photographic film. When the two lights meet they form an interference pattern on the holographic plate which looks nothing like the rose. It looks like complex rings of black and white alternating lines (see Diagram #5). The particle form of the hologram is produced when another laser is shined through the holographic film. What appears is a three-dimensional hologram image of the rose, in full color, sitting in space just in front of the film. You can walk around the rose and view it from all angles, but if you try to touch it, your hand will go right through it. It is like having a vision of a spirit with a refined body, with the spirit body standing in mid air (see Diagram # 6).

Holograms are visual expressions of the basic contradictory, wave/particle properties of light. Holograms are interesting in any study of light because they express in a larger form what is happening on the minute subatomic level. Subatomic elements are continually changing from energy to matter.

Holograms also display how subatomic elements can be interconnected. If the holographic film is cut into two pieces and then a light is shined through each piece, each portion of film will show an intact rose. The rose image is not cut in half. The entire rose is present in both pieces of film. If the film is cut into a thousand pieces, each piece will have the whole rose expressed (see Diagram # 6). In other words, every small section of the film has a memory of the whole and we don't understand how it works. There is no local spot where the image of the rose resides. The entire holographic film is interconnected. By being omnipresent on the film in the wave form, and at the same time, being a single three dimensional entity in front of the film in the particle form, the rose is infinite and finite at the same time!

A hologram is not just an isolated phenomenon. The human brain acts like a hologram. Memory is not located in individual nerve fibers. It is scattered throughout entire sections of the brain, so that any small portion of a given section of the brain contains the memory of the whole section. For example, there is a visual section of the brain that records the memory of what we see, and there is an olfactory section that records smell. Memories cannot be cut out of the brain without destroying an entire section. Even though part of a section is removed, memories stay intact. Just like every portion of a holographic film contains all the information to create an image in its particle form, every portion of each section of the brain contains all the information specific to that section of the brain to create memory. The image we see doesn't form a single smaller image in our brain, rather the image is dispersed as interference waves throughout the vision section of the brain.

Nerves in the brain are the roads on which electrical impulses travel. Nerves start as a single fiber but quickly fan out into thousands of smaller branches. These branches overlap and connect with each other. The nerves act like water in a pool, and the electrical impulses, whether visual, auditory or olfactory, act like the stones dropped in the water which form waves, causing thousands of interference patterns in the brain.

Holograms have a high capacity to store information. Just one square inch of holographic film can store over 1,500 pages of a textbook. The brain can store millions of pieces of information because it acts like a hologram. This explains why some people have photographic memories, how feelings return again and again, how we can sense pain in a leg which has been amputated, and how every sensory impression, emotion, thought or action is recorded to be played back at some future time when our life review is seen as a hologram before us.

Bohm thought that the entire universe is one big hologram, continually expressing itself in both wave and particle form. There is an interconnectedness between subatomic parts, which interchange with each other, coming in and out of existence and not being restricted to one place or time. Quantum mechanics deals with probabilities instead of certainties, stating that a certain subatomic particle has a probability of being in a certain position and having a certain velocity (speed) at any given moment. The boundaries of time and space become blurred in the small unseen world of atoms.

Bohm's work was an attempt to unite the interconnected and timeless world of the atom with the physical and time world that we are familiar with. It was an attempt to explain how one thing can be two different things. He used the known properties of holograms as an example of how the two parts of nature can be explained. Perhaps by discovering the universal connectedness of subatomic elements, scientists discovered the spiritual portion of our universe. Perhaps they have opened a small window to help us understand not only the nature of our universe but the nature of our God.

CELESTIAL HOLOGRAMS

If Bohm's speculation is correct and we do live in a holographic universe, it could help explain some of the mysteries of God. Universal holograms could be one explanation of how the ubiquitous attributes of an all-powerful God can be compatible with a glorified being who has a body. Could the grand secret of the nature of God be that he is a celestial hologram, being both infinite and finite, being the ultimate expression of matter, energy, and light? Could he be both wave and particle, energy and matter, spirit and body, everywhere and somewhere, universal yet personal, all-powerful yet intimate?

Surely God's glorified body is only one expression of his being. His being is not just a finite body with a spirit restricted to the body form. He supposedly has a spirit in the shape of his body. His spirit and intelligence could be universal, in the whole of the universe, giving life to every element throughout. In the wave form of a celestial hologram he could be omnipresent and unrestricted by time. In the particle form of that same celestial hologram he could have a glorified physical body isolated to one place. Maybe celestial life means having full access to both forms of reality. If so, the veil we are within during mortal life could be our restriction to the physical form of reality, preventing us from coming into the universal spiritual presence of God. In mortality our physical bodies are dominant over our spiritual bodies, unlike God who would have equal and full access to both spirit and matter.

The hologram is a real phenomenon. But it is speculation that our universe, and our spiritual and physical worlds might be universal holograms. However, the holographic model is exciting because it can clarify why there had to be a spiritual creation before a physical creation, why we were organized spiritually before physically, and why the world was organized in its spiritual wave form first before it was organized in its physical particle form. All matter, whether animate or inanimate, would have been organized the same way.

The holographic model can help us understand the scriptures that seem so confusing when they tell us that three Gods are one, that God is one with us, that God is in us and we in him. The three witnesses end their testimony of the Book of Mormon with these words: "And the honor be to the Father, and the Son, and the Holy Ghost, *which is one God.* Amen" (Introduction to the *Book of Mormon*, italics added). Christ said, "I and my Father are one" (John 10:30), and he also prayed, "Holy Father, keep through thine own name those whom thou has given me, that they may be one, as we are.... That they all may be one: as thou, Father art in me, and I in thee, that they also may be one in us" (John, 17:11, 21; italics added). The Godhead is one because they are one in purpose, but their oneness may be more than that. When the scriptures tell of the unity of the Godhead, maybe they are describing the unity the Godhead shares in the wave form of light, in the portion of a celestial hologram where time is not a factor and all things are part of a whole, interconnected with each other.

There is not just one giant universal hologram which includes all spiritual and physical elements of our existence. There can be innumerable holograms. In our original hologram of the rose, if the laser's position is changed so its light reflects off the rose at a different angle, a new hologram is produced. That is how our brain can learn so many things. The same nerves are used but different information (light) coming down them produces millions of different holograms. Any idea, emotion, object, smell, sound, or action can produce an individual hologram. Moving objects would produce a series of holograms like the film of a movie picture. There can even be holograms in holograms, so that one hologram may include others. There could be a hologram of spirit prison, which would not be the same as the hologram of paradise, etc. Holograms do not necessarily overlap except in a universal, celestial hologram which would include all other holograms throughout the universe.

If there is a celestial hologram our ultimate expression in the particle form could be as glorified individuals, with agency. But the other half of our beings would be shared universal light and glory, binding us eternally together with all other celestial beings. The shared portion, which includes intelligence and spirit, would be purified light and glory, fully expressed in its wave form. The universal nature of God's light which is in each of us now, gives us light and life, or we would not exist. God is in us and we are in him (D&C 88:41, 50). Just as one small section of the hologram of the rose has the whole of the rose in it, any part of the purified light of God in the wave form would contain the whole of God, and the fullness of his attributes. Any man touching, physically or spiritually, any part of the hologram of God touches the fullness of his being. "Behold, all these are kingdoms, and any man who hath seen any or the least of these hath seen God moving in his majesty and power" (D&C 88:47).

APPENDIX E

15 Billion Years Equals 6 Days
Reference # 23, Chapter Eight

The science of the big bang theory is the science of the physical earth and the creation of the physical universe. Scientists have declared the age of the universe to be around 15 billion years since the big bang. By using radioactive decay of carbon 14 as a timer, scientists tell us the earth is about 5 billion years old, and that fossils have been present on the earth for about 3.5 billion years. The chronology of the Bible, on the other hand, tells us the earth is just under 6 thousand years old since Adam and Eve fell, and that it took just six days to create the earth and the heavens. Our choices in the past to resolve this conflict have been to accept the Biblical account as an allegorical attempt to explain the unknown; to accept either the scientific time table or the religious time table, and declare the other side wrong; to accept the days of the Bible as periods of time but not 24 hour days as we know them; to give up and not resolve the problem; or to resolve that 15 billion years really does equal 6 days.

One answer to this conflict resides in the law of relativity. By 1905, physicists knew that the behavior of light and objects moving close to the speed of light was not compatible with Newton's laws of physics. Einstein's theory of special relativity addressed the new questions. In Newtonian physics, time is absolute and universal, but relativity has shown that time can be warped—expanded or reduced by motion. Each observer has his own individual reference frame of time, which never appears warped to him, and all the laws of physics are the same for each observer in his own coordinate system. It is only when one observer views another person traveling at a different speed that their two relative times become distorted and out of step. The key here is seeing the same event from one place in the universe relative to seeing the same event from another place in the universe. Time that seems so reliable and constant as we know it, really does not tick at the same rate throughout the universe. Time is constant as related to each observer; but relative to other reference frames, time is markedly variable. The faster we are moving through space the slower our clock ticks relative to other observers traveling at a slower rate. Relativity is not just a theory of science but is fact and is one of the laws of physics.

In Einstein's famous theoretical twin experiment, one twin flies in a rocket pushing the speed of light. The second twin stays on earth waiting ten years for his brother's return. When the two reunite, the rocket twin has only aged a fraction of the earth-bound twin's ten years. They both are traveling in time, but the warping of time will enable the earth-bound twin to have his ninetieth birthday years before his astronaut brother. The returning twin will also be smaller, because relative to the earthly twin, the twin racing near the speed of light will shrink. Objects contract as they approach the speed of light.

If a clock sitting on a yard stick traveling the speed of light passes a person standing on earth, the clock will tick slower and the yard stick would be shorter, relative to a clock and a yard stick on earth. It makes no sense to ask which clock is right or which yard stick is the correct length. Each is correct in its reference frame. Bodies moving close to the speed of light also show increased mass, and the closer to the speed of light, the greater the increase of mass. In our ordinary visual world this property is negligible, but at the subatomic level, electrons and protons increase their mass dozens of times as they approach the speed of light.

Not only is time warped, but space is also warped. General relativity states that gravity bends light and the more gravity there is, the more the light is bent. If there were a star hidden behind the sun, it would be possible for someone on earth to see the hidden star because as the light from the star comes into the gravitational field of the sun, the sun's gravity would bend the star's light and that warping of light would allow those on earth to see the hidden star. The star would look as if it were at the side of the sun, but in reality it would be behind the sun.

Space is not uniform or equal but is curved by gravity, depending on the distribution of matter in the universe. Not only does gravity warp space, it also slows down time, and the greater the gravity the greater time is shrunk. Time is dynamic, not absolute, fixed or universal. Time flows at different rates throughout the universe, as it is stretched, shrunk or warped by speed and gravity. The universe is not three dimensional, with time being a separate entity, but is four dimensional with the fourth dimension being a space-time continuum.

It is the relative nature of time that gives one solution to how billions of years equal 6 days. When the big bang was set off, energy and matter were in constant and rapid flux, with pure energy overpowering matter. Time and space came into existence after the big bang because time and space are related to the physical/particle phase of light and not to the spiritual/wave form of light. Who was recording the first six days of the universe and by which clock? If it was God watching the clock and watching light change into matter from the existing void, maybe the universe began from the reference frame of God and then developed millions of different time frames as solar systems developed. There are millions of reference frames (positions) throughout the universe, each traveling at different speeds and each having variable strengths of gravity. There is no common time between solar systems in the universe or between the creator and any given part of the universe, regardless of distance, size or configuration. It is impossible for one single clock to have timed all the events of the creation of the universe. There are billions of clocks keeping their own time, differing relative to each other, but all constant relative to their own time frame. If there were a clock on earth at the beginning of the big bang it could have recorded 15 billion years, and if there were a clock, with a reference frame of God while he was creating the heavens and earth, it might have rolled over twenty-four hours, six days as we know it. It is possible that the earth is both 15 billion years old and also 6 days old, plus the 6,000 years since the fall!

Gerald Schroeder, summarizes the solution this way: "According to Einstein's law of relativity, we now know it is impossible in an expanding universe to describe the elapsed time experienced during a sequence of events occurring in one part of the universe in a way that will be equal to the elapsed time for those same events when viewed from another part of the universe. The differences in motions and gravitational forces among the various galaxies, or even among the stars of a single galaxy, make the absolute passage of time a very local affair. Time differs from place to place.

"The Bible is a guidebook for mankind's passage through life and time. To instill in mankind a reverence for the physical wonders of the universe, this guide includes a description of the development that led from a void, unformed universe to a home suitable for mankind. But choosing an all-encompassing time frame to describe that span of development is nearly impossible because so many factors have an intimate and profound effect on the rate at which time passes. These include the forces of gravity within the multitude of stars that converted the primeval hydrogen and helium into elements of life, the motions of the intergalactic gases as they contracted into nebulas and then into stars, the supernovas' explosions marking the death and ultimate rebirth of the stars from which the Milky Way formed, and the mass of the Earth. The flow of time had been the one aspect of life that, until Einstein's insight, we were so erroneously certain was constant. It is unrealistic, no it is impossible, for a single clock to have timed all the ages of all the cosmic stuff of which we are composed" (Gerald Schroeder, *Genesis and the Big Bang* [New York: Bantam Books, 1990], pp. 50–51).

APPENDIX F

Note 1, Reference # 8, Chapter Ten

Throughout his life, and culminating in one of his most profound speeches, (The King Follett discourse, given during general conference, Sunday, April 7, 1844, just three months short of his martyrdom) Joseph continued to preach about our eternal nature.

"I have another subject to dwell upon, which is calculated to exalt man. . . . It is . . . the soul the mind of man the immortal spirit. Where did it come from? . . . We say that God Himself is a self-existing being . . . Who told you that man did not exist in like manner upon the same principles? Man does exist upon the same principles . . . The mind or the intelligence which man possesses is co-equal [i.e., co-eternal] with God himself. I know that my testimony is true . . . Is it logical to say that the intelligence of spirits is immortal, and yet it has a beginning? The intelligence of spirits had no beginning, neither will it have an end. That is good logic . . . Intelligence is eternal and exists upon a self-existing principle . . . The first principles of man are self-existing with God" (HC 6:310–312).

Note 2, Reference #27, Chapter Fourteen

"As revealed in one person's near-death experience: 'All through this, he kept stressing the importance of love. The places where he showed it best involved my sister; I have always been very close to her. He showed me some instances where I had been selfish to my sister, but then just as many times where I had really shown love to her and had shared with her. He pointed out to me that I should try to do things for other people, to try my best. There wasn't any accusation in any of this, though. When he came across times when I had been selfish, his attitude was only that I had been learning from them, too. He seemed very interested in things concerning knowledge, too. He kept on pointing out things that had to do with learning, and he did say that I was going to continue learning, and he said that even when he comes back for me (because by this time he had told me that I was going back) that there will always be a quest for knowledge. He said that it is a continuous process, so I got the feeling that it goes on after death. I think that he was trying to teach me, as we went through the flashbacks'" (Raymond Moody, *Life After Life* [NY: Bantam Books, 1976], pp. 67–68).

References

CHAPTER ONE

1. D&C 50:24
2. D&C 93:36, italics added
3. Acts 22:6
4. Acts 7:55
5. P of G P JS 2:16–17
6. D&C 110:3
7. Joseph Smith, Jr., et al., *History of the Church of Jesus Christ of Latter-day Saints,* edited by B. H. Roberts [Salt Lake City: Deseret Book Co., 6 vols., 1946], 2:380
8. Moses 1:5, 4
9. Moses 1:12, 13; italics added
10. Moses 1:13–16
11. Moses 1:27, 28, 37–39; italics added
12. Isaiah 33:14
13. D&C 133:40–42, 49
14. HC 6:366
15. Exodus 24:15–17
16. Moses 1:11
17. D&C 76:114–119
18. Hebrews 12:29
19. Moses 1:39
20. D&C 93:29
21. D&C 101:25, 65
22. D&C 76:7–8
23. D&C 76:92

24. D&C 88:4
25. D&C 84:24
26. D&C 88:11
27. John 1:4
28. D&C 93:29
29. D&C 88:13
30. Moroni 7:18
31. D&C 84:45, 46
32. D&C 77:4, 88:11, 45:9; 2 Corinthians 4:6
33. D&C 88:13
34. D&C 84:32
35. D&C 88:40

CHAPTER TWO

1. James Reston Jr., *Galileo* [New York: Harper-Collins, 1994], p. 283
2. 1 John 1:5
3. D&C 88:7–9
4. D&C 88:13, italics added
5. See APPENDIX A, Diagram # 1
6. There are one million nanometers in one millimeter, and there are a thousand millimeters in a meter, which is about the length of a yard.
7. D&C 88:6
8. D&C 88:7–11, italics added
9. D&C 88:13, italics added
10. D&C 88:36–39
11. See APPENDIX A, Diagram # 2
12. See APPENDIX A, Diagram # 3
13. Melvin Morse, with Paul Perry, *Transformed by the Light* [New York: Villard Books, 1992], p. 135, italics added
14. D&C 93:33
15. HC 3:387
16. HC 6:308–309
17. Parley P. Pratt, *Key to the Science of Theology* [SLC, Utah: Deseret Book, 1978 printing], pp. 26–27
18. D&C 93:29
19. Joseph Smith, HC 4:575

20. D&C 84:45
21. D&C 88:13

CHAPTER THREE

1. See APPENDIX B, The Interconnectedness of Light
2. Michael Talbot, *The Holographic Universe* [N.Y., Harper Collins, 1991], p. 38
3. Michael Talbot, *The Holographic Universe*, p. 50
4. See APPENDIX C, The Unity of Light
5. Fred Hoyle, *Frontiers of Astronomy* [New York: Harper, 1955], p. 304
6. Gary Zukav, *The Dancing Wu Li Masters* [New York: Bantam Books, 1980], p. 48
7. Brigham Young, et el. *Journal of Discourses,* 26 vols. [London and Liverpool: LDS Booksellers Depot, 1855–86], 3:277
8. JD 7:2–3
9. JD 21:234
10. D&C 88:25–26
11. D&C 131:7, see also HC 5:393
12. See APPENDIX D, Holograms and the Nature of Light and God
13. Ether 3:6, italics added
14. Ether 3:13
15. D&C 38:1–2

CHAPTER FOUR

1. Moses 1:33, 38
2. D&C 88:47
3. D&C 88:13
4. D&C 93:36
5. D&C 93:35
6. HC 6:308, italics added
7. D&C 88:41, 50
8. *The Seer* II p. 227, italics added
9. D&C 38:2
10. Moses 1:6
11. D&C 130:7
12. D&C 93:29

13. D&C 93:36
14. D&C 88:66
15. D&C 93:24
16. Alma 7:13
17. Isaiah 46:9, 10
18. HC 2:12
19. Moses 1:31, 27–29
20. Moses 1:35
21. Moses 1:10
22. Gen. 17:1
23. D&C 61:1
24. D&C 88:7–10
25. D&C 88:13
26. HC 4:78
27. D&C 88:12–13, 36–38
28. II Nephi 2:13
29. I Nephi 9:6
30. Moses 7:63; D&C 38:4
31. Ether 3:4
32. D&C 19:3
33. Alma 12:15
34. Alma 12:15
35. D&C 84:102
36. D&C 109:77
37. Moses 6:61
38. D&C 88:12, 13, 45
39. Abraham 3:4
40. D&C 88:42–44
41. D&C 88:42, 44
42. Alma 40:8
43. Revelation 10:4–6
44. D&C 88:110
45. JD 13:77
46. Neal Maxwell, *All These Things Shall Give Thee Experience* [SLC: Deseret Book, 1979], p. 11
47. Moses 1:39
48. I John 4:5

49. I John 4:16
50. I Nephi 8:12
51. I Nephi 11:22
52. Alma 19:6
53. II Nephi, 11:22
54. D&C 18:16
55. Alma 36:24
56. D&C 18:13
57. Moses 7:33
58. Moses 7:41
59. John A. Widtsoe, *Conference Report*, 1943, April p. 38
60. D&C 93:16, 19
61. Matt. 10:39

CHAPTER FIVE

1. Raymond A. Moody, *The Light Beyond* [New York: Bantam Books, 1989], pp. 88–91
2. Duane Crowther, *Life Everlasting* [Salt Lake City: Bookcraft, 1967]
3. Arvin S. Gibson, *Glimpses of Eternity* [Bountiful, Utah: Horizon Publishing, 1992]
4. Brent and Wendy Top, *Beyond Death's Door* [Salt Lake City: Bookcraft, 1993]
5. George G. Ritchie, *My Life After Dying* [Norfolk, VA: Hampton Roads Publishing Co., 1991], p. 16
6. Kenneth Ring, *Heading Toward Omega* [New York: Quill, 1985], p. 66
7. Moody, *The Light Beyond*, p. 12–13
8. Carol Zaleski, *Otherworld Journeys* [New York: Oxford University press, 1981], p. 125, italics in original
9. *Messenger and Advocate*, October 1834, 1:14–15, see footnote P of GP JS
10. Arvin Gibson, *Glimpses of Eternity,* p. 300
11. 3 Nephi 17:15–17
12. 3 Nephi 17:24–25, italics added
13. Howard Storm, International *IANDS* Conference, August, 16–19, 1990, p. 9

14. Kenneth Ring, *Heading Toward Omega* [New York: Quill, 1985], p. 197
15. Kenneth Ring, *Heading Toward Omega*, p. 196
16. Arvin Gibson, *Glimpses of Eternity*, p. 223
17. Arvin Gibson, *Glimpses of Eternity*, p. 223
18. Raymond Moody, *Reflections on Life After Life* [New York: Bantam Books, 1977], pp. 9–11
19. Carol Zaleski, *Otherworld Journeys*, p. 117
20. Raymond Moody, M.D., *Life After Life*, p. 48
21. Raymond Moody, M.D., *The Light Beyond*, p. 18
22. Kenneth Ring, *Life After Death* [New York: Quill, 1982], p. 98
23. George G. Ritchie, *Return from Tomorrow* [Old Tappen, New Jersey: Spire Books, 1978], p. 45
24. John 14:27
25. Emanuel Swedenborg, *Heaven and Hell*, Translated by George F. Dole, 58th printing [New York: Swedenborg Foundation, 1990], pp. 38–39
26. Margot Grey, *Return From Death* [London: Arkana, 1987], pp. 53–54
27. Kenneth Ring, *Heading Toward Omega* [New York: Quill, 1985], pp. 40, 50
28. I Cor. 13:13
29. Arvin Gibson, *Glimpses of Eternity*, p. 293
30. Margot Grey, *Return From Death* [London: Arkana, 1987], p. 53
31. George G. Ritchie, *Return from Tomorrow*, pp. 48–49

CHAPTER SIX

1. D&C 93:4
2. D&C 132:5, 21; 130:20, 21
3. Moses 4:2, italics added
4. III Nephi 11:11
5. Ps. 89:27; see also D&C 93:21
6. Abraham 3:19, italics added
7. Ether 3:16, see Moroni's comment, Ether 3:17
8. Bruce R. McConkie, *The Promised Messiah* [Salt Lake City: Deseret Book Co., 1978], pp. 48–49
9. Moses 4:2

10. Rev. 13:8
11. Heb. 5:9
12. Abraham 3:24
13. John 17:5
14. D&C 76:13
15. Matt. 28:18
16. D&C 88:4–6, italics added
17. D&C 93:16–17, italics added
18. JST Luke 10:23
19. John 14:10–11, italics added
20. D&C 93:3–4
21. Mosiah 15:1–5
22. D&C 29:1, 42
23. D&C 49:5, 28
24. *Lectures on Faith,* #5
25. D&C 88:11
26. Pratt, *Key to the Science of Theology,* p. 25
27. D&C 88:50
28. D&C 18:34–35
29. Orson Pratt, JD 17:327
30. D&C 84:45–46
31. D&C 11:12–13
32. JD 8:205
33. Ether 3:14, italics added
34. Heb. 1:3

CHAPTER SEVEN

1. Joseph Smith, *Teachings,* p. 190
2. Alma 11:44, italics added
3. D&C 130:22
4. D&C 93:4
5. D&C 130:22
6. Gen. 17:1
7. John 8:12
8. Moses 5:9
9. III Nephi 28:11

10. I Cor. 12:3
11. Jacob 7:11–12
12. D&C 20:27–28
13. John 15:26
14. John 16:13–14, italics added
15. D&C 84:45
16. D&C 84:45, 46
17. D&C 93:26
18. D&C 88:66
19. John 14:16–17
20. John 16:13
21. Brigham Young, JD 1:50
22. Ether 3:15–16
23. D&C 84:45, 88:6–13
24. Joseph Smith, *Teachings,* p. 328
25. Moroni 10:4–5
26. D&C 42:17
27. D&C 39:6
28. D&C 31:11
29. D&C 50:14
30. D&C 28:1
31. D&C 75:27
32. D&C 79:2
33. D&C 90:11
34. D&C 90:14
35. D&C 90:15
36. D&C 8:2–3
37. D&C 130:23
38. Ex. 31:3
39. Acts 1:8
40. Acts 2:17
41. I Cor. 12:8
42. Heb. 2:4
43. I Cor. 12:9
44. John 14:26
45. D&C 20:77–79
46. D&C 39:6

47. Joseph Smith, *Teachings,* p. 199
48. D&C 35:6
49. John 3:5
50. Alma 13:12
51. III Nephi 27:20
52. III Nephi 11:35
53. Mosiah 4:3
54. Matt. 3:11
55. Isaiah 33:14

CHAPTER EIGHT

1. Genesis 1:2
2. Genesis 1:3, 4
3. Isaiah 45:7
4. Abraham 4:4
5. Moses 1:35, 38
6. Orson Pratt, *The Seer* II #4, April 1854, p. 248–249, italics added
7. Mark 5:25–34
8. Moses 1:33, 38
9. HC 3:387
10. HC 6:308–309
11. D&C 93:29, 33
12. B. H. Roberts, *The Way, The Truth, The Life*, pp. 60–61
13. HC 6:308, italics added
14. Abraham 4:1
15. Abraham 4:7
16. Abraham 4:18
17. Abraham 4:31
18. Genesis 1:10, 12, 18, 21, 25, 31
19. Abraham 4:31
20. Gerald L. Schroeder, *Genesis and the Big Bang*, Bantam Books, New York, 1990, p. 97
21. Moses 3:4–7
22. Isaac Newton, *Mathematical Principle of Natural Philosophy*
23. See APPENDIX E, 15 Billion Years Equal 6 Days
24. D&C 88:42–44, italics added

25. Abraham 3:6–10, italics added
26. Abraham 5:13
27. *The Mormon*, August 29, 1857
28. TS III February 1, 1842, p. 672
29. D&C 84:45, italics added
30. Moses 1:30
31. Moses 1:32–33, 38; italics added
32. John 1:1–5, see also D&C 93:8–9
33. Moses 2:1, 5; italics added
34. D&C 88:66, italics added
35. III Ne. 9:15
36. Col. 1:16–17
37. Mosiah 3:5, 8
38. Abr. 4:18, 31
39. Moses 1:30–33, 38
40. D&C 88:12–13
41. D&C 88:36–38, 42–45

CHAPTER NINE

1. John 17:5
2. I Nephi 11:16–18, 20–2
3. John 17:5
4. D&C 88:6
5. I Nephi 11:21
6. Luke 1:35
7. Bruce R. McConkie, *The Promised Messiah* [SLC: Deseret Book, 1978], p. 467
8. D&C 93:6–11 italic added
9. John 4:25–26, italics added
10. John 8:42, 56–58; italics added
11. John 10:24, 30, 32–36; italics added
12. JST John 1:19
13. John 8:12
14. John 14:6
15. John 6:51
16. John 11:25

References

17. B. H. Roberts, *The Truth, The Way, The Life*, p. 479
18. Matt. chapter 5, 6
19. Matt. 6:9–13
20. I Nephi 11:28, italics added
21. Alma 9:26
22. Mark 1:22–28, 30–31, 34, 39, 40–43; 2:1–3, 5
23. Mark 8:1–9
24. John 11:43–44
25. John 5:19
26. Luke 2:49
27. Moses 1:39
28. Mosiah 15:7
29. Matt. 26:38
30. D&C 76:41
31. Moses 5:57
32. Moses 7:47
33. Heb. 7:26
34. Heb. 4:15
35. John 5:26
36. John 19:30
37. Alma 34:10, 12
38. Mark 15:34
39. D&C 19:18
40. D&C 133:50
41. Brigham Young, JD 3:206, italics added
42. D&C 18:11
43. II Nephi 9:21
44. Isaiah 53:10–11, italics added
45. John 1:14
46. Heb. 2:17–18
47. John Taylor, *The Meditation and Atonement* [SLC: Stevens & Wallis, Inc., 1950 printing] p. 142, italics added
48. John 17:3–5
49. Heb. 5:8–9
50. Alma 7:11–12, italics added
51. III Nephi 27:14
52. Heb. 10:11

53. D&C 88:6
54. D&C 93:11, 16
55. III Nephi 15:9
56. D&C 88:13
57. Alma 42:10–18
58. D&C 19:16–18
59. Alma 42:23–24
60. D&C 88:6, 37–38
61. D&C 88:40–41, italics added
62. D&C 88:38–39
63. D&C 88:40
64. Eccl. 11:1
65. D&C 93:12–14, 16; italics added
66. Moroni 7:47
67. I John 4:16
68. D&C 110:2–3, italics added
69. D&C 76:23–24
70. III Nephi 11:11, 14
71. II Thess. 1:7
72. Psalm 97:1, 2, 4–6; italics added
73. II Peter 3:10
74. D&C 63:20, 21
75. Matt. 6:10
76. D&C 45:48
77. Joseph Smith I 1:36
78. Matt. 25:31

CHAPTER TEN

1. D&C 93:21, 23; italics added
2. D&C 93:29
3. D&C 84:45, 46
4. D&C 88:40
5. D&C 93:26
6. HC 3:387
7. HC 4:79
8. HC 6:310–312, italics added; see APPENDIX F, Note 1

9. D&C 93:30, 31
10. BY as quoted in *The Resurrection*, SLC, 1884, p. 3
11. BY, JD 3:277
12. Abr. 3:18
13. B. H. Roberts, *The Truth, the Way, the Life*, pp. 78, 80, 81
14. II Nephi 2:13
15. D&C 93:30
16. D&C 88:36–38
17. Abr. 3:22
18. Abr. 3:26
19. HC 6:311, 312
20. Brigham Young, JD 7:2–3
21. D&C 93:21
22. B. H. Roberts, *The Way, the Truth, the Life*, p. 250
23. D&C 93:29
24. Acts 17:29
25. Brigham Young, JD 1:50, 4:216, 6:31
26. Ether 3:15–16
27. D&C 77:2
28. Parley P. Pratt, JD 1:7–8, italics added
29. Moses 3:5
30. B. H. Roberts, *The Truth, The Way, The Life*, p. 256–257
31. Abr. 3:26
32. D&C 93:25
33. Moses 1:33–34
34. Rev. 14:6–7
35. Rev. 13:8
36. Heb. 13:20
37. Titus 1:2
38. HC 6:308
39. Moses 4:1
40. Joseph Smith, HC 6:314
41. Moses 4:2, italics added
42. Abr. 3:27
43. D&C 93:25
44. Jacob 7:18, 19
45. D&C 76:25–26

46. Rev. 12:7–8
47. Luke 10:18
48. D&C 93:31, italics added
49. Rev. 12:4
50. Joseph Fielding Smith, *Doctrines of Salvation*, Vol I , [SLC: Bookcraft, 1954], pp. 56–57, italics in original text
51. Moses 1:39
52. Nephi 2:25
53. D&C 93:33–35, italics added
54. As quoted in the *Deseret News* XIV, Aug. 23, 1865, pp. 372–374
55. D&C 29:31–32
56. Abr. 3:26
57. D&C 93:29
58. D&C 93:29
59. D&C 93:36

CHAPTER ELEVEN

1. Job 38:6–7
2. D&C 1:31
3. II Nephi 2:11, 13
4. II Nephi 2:23
5. II Nephi, 2:13
6. B. H. Roberts, *The Truth , the Way, the Life*, p. 334
7. Abr. 3:18; D&C 93:29, 30
8. Gen. 1:1–3; Isa. 45:7
9. Abr. 3:25–26
10. D&C 29:36, 39–40
11. Moses 2:28
12. Moses 3:16–17
13. Moses 3:17
14. Rev. 13:8
15. Moses 4:10, 11
16. Moses 4:28
17. D&C 29:46–47
18. Moses 5:10–11

19. Joseph Fielding Smith, *Doctrine of Salvation* [SLC, Bookcraft, 1954], p. 114, italics in the original text
20. D&C 29:36–43
21. Gen. 3:22–24
22. John 8:43
23. D&C 88:48–49
24. Matt. 25:14–30
25. I John 2:9, 4:20
26. John 3:20
27. III Nephi 13:22–23
28. D&C 10:21, italics added
29. D&C 29:45, italics added
30. I Nephi 17:45, italics added
31. D&C 93:39
32. D&C 88:34, 35
33. II Nephi 15:20
34. D&C 93:37
35. Ether 4:15
36. II Nephi 26:29, italics added
37. II Nephi 2:7
38. Luke 18:14

CHAPTER TWELVE

1. Alma 42:7
2. D&C 29:42
3. Moses 5:7, 6:52
4. Moses 6:64
5. I Nephi 8:23
6. I Nephi 8:10
7. I Nephi 11:22, 25
8. I Nephi 11:7, 32–33; italics added
9. Alma 5:34
10. Mosiah 26:23
11. Alma 39:15
12. Alma 11:40
13. Alma 12:15

14. D&C 88:11, 67
15. D&C 84:46
16. I Nephi 8:35
17. Ether 12:32
18. II Nephi 31:20
19. Moroni 7:41–44, italics added
20. Alma 34:10–14
21. D&C 88:41
22. Moses 7:47
23. Moses 6:53–54
24. Alma 36:16, 19–20
25. Enos 1:5
26. Isaiah 22:23–24
27. Rom 3:23
28. Alma 12:15
29. D&C 20:72–79
30. Mosiah 14:10–11; D&C 25:1
31. D&C 88:13
32. John 8:12; D&C 10:70
33. D&C 88:50
34. Stephen E. Robinson, *Following Christ* [SLC: Deseret Book, 1995], pp. 4–5, italics in the original
35. D&C 88:38–39
36. D&C 93:38
37. II Nephi 2:5–8
38. Gal 2:16, 3:11
39. D&C 20:30
40. Matt. 11:28–30, italics added
41. Numbers 21:7–9
42. Alma 37:46
43. Isaiah 1:18
44. Stephen A. Robinson, *Believing Christ* [SLC: Deseret Book, 1992], p. 8, italics in the original
45. II Nephi 4:17–20
46. Mosiah 4:3
47. Alma 36:18–20, italics added
48. D&C 84:102

49. John 14:27, 16:33
50. Heb. 5:8, 9
51. Matt. 5:45
52. Viktor E. Frankl, *Man's Search for Meaning* [New York: Washington Square Press, 1984], pp. 87, 86
53. Frankl, *Man's Search*, p. 88
54. Psalms 55:22
55. Isaiah 10:27
56. Jacob 4:7
57. Ether 12:27
58. II Nephi 2:25

CHAPTER THIRTEEN

1. Luke 15:20–24
2. Enos 1:9
3. I Nephi 8:11–12, italics added
4. Matt. 5:14
5. Mosiah 18:9
6. Mosiah 18:11
7. Mosiah 4:26
8. D&C 64:34
9. Mosiah 4:27, italics added
10. Matt. 25:24–30
11. D&C 93:12–13, 16
12. Eccl 11:1
13. Matt. 16:25
14. D&C 93:20
15. D&C 50:22
16. D&C 46:11
17. Matt. 5:16
18. Hel. 3:35
19. Brigham Young, JD 11:237
20. Moroni 10:20, 21
21. D&C 88:125
22. Moroni 10:32–33
23. III Nephi 27:20

24. John 6:51, 53–58
25. Moses 6:59–60; D&C 88:20
26. John A. Widtsoe, *Priesthood and Church Government* [SLC: Deseret Book, 1961], p. 35
27. Joseph Smith, *Teachings of the Prophet Joseph Smith* [SLC: Deseret Book, 1968], p. 167, italics added
28. Joseph Smith, *Teachings of the Prophet Joseph Smith*, p. 157; Abraham 1:2
29. Widtsoe, *Priesthood and Church Government*, p. 348
30. D&C 84:19–22, italics added
31. John 6:63
32. Mosiah 5:15
33. Joseph Smith, HC 5:423, italics added
34. HC 5:427
35. HC 5:423
36. D&C 43:16
37. Matt 16:19; D&C 132:46
38. D&C 88:40
39. D&C 128:11–12, italics in the original
40. Alma 7:12
41. Ether 12:27–28
42. D&C 88:124–125
43. D&C 50:26
44. D&C 121:41, 42, 45
45. Moroni 7:47

CHAPTER FOURTEEN

1. III Nephi 12:47–48
2. Matt. 5:48
3. John 11:43
4. Matt. 8:3
5. Matt. 8:2
6. Rom 8:17
7. Act 17:29
8. D&C 93:19–20
9. Ephesians 4:13

10. Kenneth Ring, *Heading Toward Omega* [NY: Quill, 1985], p. 40
11. George G. Ritchie, Jr. *Return From Tomorrow* [N.J., Spire Books, Fleming H. Revell Co.: Old Tappen, 1978], p. 49
12. Bruce R. McConkie, *Mormon Doctrine* [SLC: Bookcraft, 1966], p. 97
13. II Nephi 30:17
14. Orson Pratt, JD 2:239
15. Kenneth Ring, *Heading Toward Omega* [NY: Quill, 1985], pp. 69–69
16. George G. Ritchie, *Return From Tomorrow*, pp. 49–50
17. P. M. H. Atwater, *Coming Back to Life* [NY: Dodd, Mead & Co., 1988], p. 36
18. JST Matt. 7:2, 3
19. Matt. 5:7
20. D&C 121:45
21. Arvin Gibson, *Glimpses of Eternity*, p. 294
22. George G. Ritchie, *Return From Tomorrow*, p. 54–55
23. D&C 88:109, italics added
24. D&C 137:5–9
25. Alma 41:3–5
26. D&C 2:1
27. Raymond Moody, *Life After Life* [NY: Bantam Books, 1976], pp. 67–68, italics added; see APPENDIX F, Notes, #2
28. Arvin Gibson, *Glimpses of Eternity*, p. 324
29. D&C 130:18–19
30. D&C 64:34
31. HC 4:588
32. D&C 88:7–13
33. Joseph Smith, HC 5:387–389
34. John 14:15–18, 21, 23; italics added
35. D&C 88:3–5
36. Joseph Smith, HC 3:380–381
37. Ether 3:13
38. D&C 129:1, 3
39. D&C 88:68
40. Joseph Smith, HC 1:283–284
41. D&C 76:114–117, italics added

CHAPTER FIFTEEN

1. Moses 3:9
2. Joseph Smith, HC V p. 61
3. D&C 29:31–33
4. *Times and Seasons* III February 1, 1842, p. 672
5. Orson Pratt, JD 21:233–234
6. D&C 76:63
7. P of GP Articles of Faith 10
8. D&C 88:25–26
9. Psalm 97:3–6
10. D&C 101:24–25
11. D&C 63:20–21
12. Moses 7:48, 49, 59, 61
13. D&C 101:32–34
14. Joseph Smith, *Teachings of the Prophet Joseph Smith* [Deseret Book: SLC, 1968], p. 181
15. D&C 130:6–8
16. D&C 130:9–10
17. D&C 33:17–18
18. D&C 45:44
19. D&C 29:11
20. D&C 65:5
21. D&C 130:1
22. D&C 45:59
23. D&C 88:104
24. Rev. 22:11
25. Rev. 21:23
26. D&C 76:63–65, 70
27. D&C 88:34
28. D&C 88:28–29, italics added
29. D&C 88:20–21
30. D&C 76:63, 58–60, 62, 69–70; italics added
31. Carol Zaleski, *Otherworld Journeys* [NY: Oxford University Press, 1987], p. 126
32. Margot Grey, *Return from Death* [London: Arkana, 1987], p. 51
33. Vital Sign, IANDS, Vol xvi, Num 4, Fall 1997, p. 6

34. Kenneth Ring, *Heading Toward Omega* [NY: Quill, 1985], p. 66
35. Charles Flynn, *After the Beyond* [Englewood Cliffs, NJ: Prentice-Hall, 1986], p. 12
36. D&C 93:20
37. D&C 88:107
38. Phil. 3:21
39. II Cor. 3:18
40. Psalms 82:6
41. D&C 132:20
42. D&C 93:28
43. D&C 84:38
44. D&C 76:95–96
45. John 17:21–23
46. D&C 93:19–20, 88:3–4
47. D&C 107:18–19
48. D&C 88:68
49. D&C 76:6–10
50. D&C 88:67
51. D&C 88:49
52. D&C 93:28
53. Moses 6:61
54. Mosiah 4:3
55. Moroni 10:32–33
56. D&C 50:24, 88:67
57. Isaiah 33:14
58. D&C 35:21
59. John 10:10
60. D&C 88:49–50
61. Moses 6:67–68, italics added
62. D&C 88:41, 50
63. III Nephi 19:29, italics added
64. D&C 88:6–11
65. D&C 88:11–13
66. D&C 88:41
67. C. S. Lewis, *The Weight of Glory and other Addresses*, "Is Theology Poetry," Revised and expanded edition [NY: Macmillan, 1980], p. 92
68. III Nephi 28:10

Index

A

Abraham, 57, 58, 85
    rejoiced to see Christ's day, 91
    saw Adam and Even in Garden before they tasted forbidden fruit, 83
Adam, 111
Adam and Eve, 117
    faced opposition of good & evil, joy & sorrow, pleasure & pain, 136
    fall of ... precipitated a time change, 83
    lost their innocence, 125
    Only Begotten Son first great hope of light to, 136
added glory of God, 41
added upon, 115
agency, 106, 124
    innate of our intelligences, 112
agency and opposition
    maintained in the fall of Adam and Eve, 123
agency, inherent, 107
    difference between things which act and things that are acted on, 107
Alma, 35, 37, 42, 139, 144, 145
Atonement, 64, 94, 117, 140
    all mankind lost without, 68
    Christ's ... was culmination of premortal plans, 95
    Christ's voluntary release of all his light, 96
    consequences for Christ, 97
    denying the power of light of Christ's, 128
    descent into hell gave innocent ... power to carry us back up, 96
    God the Father withdrew his Spirit and cast a veil over Christ, 96
    laws of justice and mercy are both fully expressed through, 99
    light of hope, 135
    light of the ... is distributed across humanity, 144
    sacrifice was infinite, 96
    six important things accomplished through the, 97
    sorrow of the, 97
    suffering, 146
    without ... justice demands we pay for our sins by loss of light, 99

B

B. H. Roberts, 79, 93, 107, 110, 121
baptism
    by fire brings sanctification, 73
    means being sanctified by the Holy Ghost, 73
    new birth into the family of Christ, 141
    our signature on the contract, 141
baptized
    when we are ..., Christ gives us spiritual life, 141
be ye therefore perfect
    wonderful commandment and promise, 165
beginning
    and end, 36
being made perfect in one, 186
Big Bang, 75
    a reorganization, 80
black holes
    light-destroying machines, 114
bodies of light, 181
body, 10
Brigham Young, 25, 40, 63, 70, 96, 106, 107
brother of Jared, 28, 29, 37, 57
Bruce R. McConkie, 58, 90

C

C. S. Lewis, 188
celestial glory, 30, 179, 182
    promise of Jesus Christ, 6
    two births into, 116
Celestial Kingdom, 5, 171
    light and glory of the, 185
charity, 151, 157
    the pure love of Christ, 163
    faith, hope, and ... bring us to full light of Christ, 138
    love unfeigned, 162
    the pure love of Christ, 101

clouds of heaven
  Jesus will come in ..., clothed with power and great glory, 180
Comforter, 69, 173
compassion, 7, 16
compound in one, 121
condescension of God, 90
conscience, 7
council of the Gods, 112
courses of heavens and earth are fixed, 86
creation, 75
  Abraham's account, 80
  beginning of ordered light, 77
  By mine Only Begotten I created these things, 84
  energy and matter were in a fluid stage and disorganized in, 76
  no creation out of nothing—ex nihilo, 79

D

darkness, 3, 131
  and evil are absence of good and light, 140
  as eternal as light, 121
  attempting to obtain light through, 113
  gravity produces, 114
  must be removed from us so we can be added upon, 178
  of perdition, 110
  tree of death, 124
  wages of Satan, 132
David Bohm, 24
death
  Christ died both a spiritual and a physical death, 96
despair, 136
dichotomy of light, 18

E

earth, 80
  a living principle following law, 26
  abides the law of a celestial kingdom, 178
  in sanctified state will be a Urim and Thummim to inhabitants, 179
  must have its corruptible elements removed, 178
  rolls upon her wings, 86
  sanctified state like a sea of glass and fire, 180
  shall die, 26
  shall pass away, 78, 79
  will be rolled back to presence of God after millennium, 179
Eastward in Eden, 117
Edwin Hubble, 75
Einstein, 12, 19
electromagnetic
  energy, 12
  force, 12
  spectrum, 14, 15
electromagnetic spectrum
  but small part of God's light, 15
  energy, 15
  intelligence, 15
  knowledge, 15
  laws, 15
  life, 15
  mercy, 15
  truth, 15
electromagnetism, 16
electron, 18
electrons
  interconnected, 24
  not independent from universe, 28
elements, 20
  are eternal, 79, 116
  have existence from time God has existed, 19
  in which dwells all glory, 33
  intelligence, spirit, matter, ..., law all variations of light, 20
  intelligence, spirit, matter, ..., law have diff. properties, 20
  not a particle of ... not filled with life, 25
  omnipresent, 27
empathic experience with Christ, 147
empathy
  may feel ... when other's energy cleaves to our energy, 148
energy, 14-16, 19, 30
  /matter, 21
  phase of light is the spirit, 59
energy and matter
  two forms of same thing, 19
Enoch, 42, 178
Enos, 152
equity, 93
eternal life
  to know God the Father and Jesus Christ, 146
Eve
  eyes were opened after being beguiled by Satan, 125

evening until morning, 80
everlasting burnings, 4, 49, 73, 186
    Almighty God dwells in eternal fire, 4
evil and darkness
    are absence of good and light, 140
ex nihilo
    no creation out of nothing, 79

F

faith
    empowers us to move toward light, 141
    hope, ..., and charity bring us to full light of Christ, 138
fall
    of Adam and Eve set stage for our journey toward added light, 123
    separation of all things culminated when Adam and Eve fell, 77
fire, 49, 102
first estate, 111
Firstborn, 105
forbidden fruit, 123
force, 11
Fred Hoyle, 24
fullness, 184
    of the Father added upon us, 185
fullness of joy, 188

G

Galileo, 9
gamma rays, 13
Gary Zukav, 25
George Ritchie, 170
Gerald Schroeder, 81
Gethsemane, 95
Gift of Holy Ghost, 71
giving and receiving, 155
glory, 1, 5, 16, 36, 38, 43, 59, 62
    added upon our heads forever and ever, 117
    all people shall see God's, 178
    all the people see Christ's, 103
    of God is intelligence, 2
    of God is truth, 34
God, 1
    Almighty dwells in eternal fire, 4
    created all things spiritually, 110
    is a consuming fire, 5
    is light, 1, 10
    is love, 41
    is omnipresent, 28
    is perfect intelligence, 35
    not responsible for consequences of those who love darkness, 122
    reveals his glory through love, mercy, power, and knowledge, 32
    used his power to separate light into its two forms, 81
God the Father, 1, 40, 43, 59, 60, 94, 98, 185, 188
    has a body of flesh and bones; the Son also, 67
    his light is his love, 1
    is both spirit and matter, 31
    is love, 1
    is omnipotent, 36
    is omnipresent, 33
    is omniscient, 34
    is perfect, 165
    my work and my glory, 3
    power love, mercy justice of, 37
    shared his glory and light with his Firstborn, 90
God's light
    is law, 36
God's omnipresence
    includes all time, 34
God's word, 84
    by power of ... matter obeyed and light was organized, 85
God's work
    is glory, 41
gods, they shall be, 185
God's glory, 3
God's light
    in physical form can be compared to particle form of light, 38
gospel of Jesus Christ
    is gospel of light, 10
grace, 91, 93, 101
    for grace, 101, 155
    light of sanctification, 154
    there is no rule on how to give, 155
gravity, 12, 82
    acts as the opposite of light, 113
    produces darkness, 114

H

heart, 10
Heavenly Parents, 40-42, 116, 159, 184, 188
holy
    we become ... when baptized by fire, 158
Holy Ghost, 5

beareth record of Father and Son, 68
brings joy, remission of sins, and peace, 73
called Spirit of the Lord, 70
come after we receive testimony of Jesus Christ, 72
comes after we are baptized by water, 72
comes by laying on of hands, 73
Comforter, 69-71
fell upon Adam, 68
gift of, 71
guides into all truth, 69
need presence of ... to gain knowledge, 72
need presence of ... to gain miracles, 72
need presence of ... to gain power, 72
need presence of ... to gain prophecy, 72
need presence of ... to gain understanding, 72
need presence of ... to gain visions, 72
need presence of ... to gain wisdom, 72
need presence of ... to gain wonders, 72
one with the Father and Christ; his light is their light, 67
part of Godhead, 67
receives what is Father's and Son's and delivers it unto us, 69
Spirit of Truth, 69, 70
Testator, 67-69
testifies of Jesus Christ, 68
touches our spirits, 71
Holy Spirit of Promise, 174
hope
comes from experiencing the light of Christ, 139
faith, ..., and charity bring us to full light of Christ, 138
in infinite nature of Atonement, 138
is based on choosing to see the light of Christ, 137

I

innocent
every spirit of man was ... in the beginning, 143
keeping law of gospel makes us ... through accepting Atonement, 142
we become ... when baptized by water, 158
intelligence, 7, 20, 34, 64, 107
..., spirit, matter, elements, law all variations of light, 20
..., spirit, matter, elements, law have diff. properties, 20
(the light of truth) not created or made, 79, 105
cleaves unto intelligence, 106
is eternal, 106
is truth, our eternal conscience, 34
light of truth not created or made, 5
was once organized with energy, the wave form of light, 29
whatever principle of ... we attain in life will rise with us, 172
intelligences, 42, 43
are infinite, 108
are light, 20
to be added upon, 108
interference, patterns of, 17
interrelated
light, energy, mass, force, work, power, 11
Isaac Newton, 26
Isaiah, 4

J

Jesus Christ , 1, 28, 40, 49, 55, 61, 102
"I am the Father and the Son", 64
became God the Savior by being only begotten of Father in flesh, 90
(Jehovah) spoke and elements came rushing together, 78
accepted all conditions of the Father's plan, 58
as Father, 62
as father with his Father, 60
as Savior, 111
Atonement of ... was culmination of premortal plans, 95
became God the Creator by inheritance, 90
began his final journey to atone for our sins, 89
began to assume eternal glory when born, 57
Beloved and Chosen from the beginning, 57
business was to glorify his Father, 94
call to all the world, "I am God! Follow me.", 93
casting our lot with, 138
celestial glory is promise of, 6
celestial glory through, 58

comprehending the purity of his Father's love, 55
created heavens and earth, 85
Creator of all things from the beginning, 85
did nothing of himself, 94
died both a spiritual and a physical death, 96
enlightens eyes, 15
entire spectrum of light was centered in, 95
entire spectrum of light was set upon cross to be sacrificed, 95
Father declared ... must have his trials as well as others, 96
firstborn in premortal world, 55, 57, 109
full of grace and truth, 91
fullness of his Father's glory, 55
gave us physical life, 141
gives life, 11
gives light, 15
gives us spiritual life when we are baptized, 141
glory of his Father, 56
governs all things through laws of justice, mercy, and love, 99
his light is law, 99
his love feeds our souls, 94
I am the Son of God, 92
immortal and mortal Christ descended below all things, 97
in all things, 11, 14
in physical form of elements, ... an individual with agency, 60
in spirit form of light, one with the Father, 60
in the beginning with the Father, 105
increases his glory as he gives us glory of celestial kingdom, 187
is light in sun and stars, 11
is love, 1
is power of God, 11
is the Father, 70
life on earth, 91
made perfect in, 186
more intelligent than all others, 57
obedience to his Father, 58
obedience to what was eternal, 56
offered himself a sacrifice for sin, 133
Only Begotten of the Father, 55, 91
Only Begotten Son from beginning, 58
people picked up stones to kill ... because message was clear, 91
performed his mission by obedience, 94
physically separate from his Father, 67
quickens understanding, 15
received all glory and power through obedience, 64
Redeemer of the world, 91
Savior, 57, 65
Second Comforter, 6, 58, 173
Second Coming of, 103
shared light and glory of his Father, 60
Son is the Father, 60
sons and daughters of, 64
Spirit of truth, 105, 106
suffered the pain of all men, 96
the Creator, 64
the Father, 67
the light of truth, 59
two parts to his being, Father and Son, 60
will come in clouds of heaven, clothed with power & great glory, 180
Word that was made flesh, 97
John, 60, 90, 101, 102
connectedness of Father and Son, 60
in the beginning the Word was, 90
saw Christ's glory in the beginning, 90
John A. Widtsoe, 42
John the Revelator, 40
Joseph Fielding Smith, 126
Joseph Smith, 2, 4-6, 11, 14, 16, 19, 20, 26, 27, 32, 33, 35, 36, 40, 48, 58, 60, 61, 71, 72, 79, 80, 86, 90, 102, 106, 130, 161, 171, 175, 179
joy, 43, 186
shall be full, 188
we receive ... by giving love, 41
judge
wisdom to, 98
judgment, 7, 169
accomplished by how much light each of us comprehends, 100
our desire for goodness is what is judged, 171
reveals light of love and light of knowledge we have gained, 172
justice, 16, 30, 38, 99
justification
being declared innocent because Christ is innocent, 142
through Christ, 156

through grace of our Lord and Savior, Jesus Christ, 143
justified
    no man is ... by law in the sight of God, 143

K

Kenneth Ring, 167
King Benjamin, 85, 153
kingdom
    every ... is given a law, 36, 101
knowledge, 7, 32, 43, 62, 107, 125, 172
    truth is, 35

L

law, 16, 20, 34
    every kingdom is given a, 36, 101
    intelligence, spirit, matter, elements, ... have diff properties, 20
    intelligence, spirit, matter, elements, ... variations of light, 20
    keeping ... of gospel makes us innocent through the Atonement, 142
    no man is justified by ... in the sight of God, 143
law of Christ
    be justified & sanctified through baptism & grace; sealed to him, 182
    of light and love, 101
laws
    and conditions of our individual kingdoms vary, 107
Lehi, 37, 107, 120
life, 7, 34
    in all matter, 24, 25
    not a particle of element not filled with, 25
light, 1, 16, 19
    ... energy and energy a form of matter, 20
    added upon our intelligences, 109
    all things are reproved by, 129
    attempting to obtain ... through darkness, 113
    basic function of ... is to be given away, 43
    bodies of, 181
    both wave and particle at same moment, so should it be with God, 38
    cleaves unto light, 100, 101, 106
    dichotomy of, 17
    gives life to all things, 86
    intelligence, spirit, matter, elements, law all variations of, 20
    is energy, 11, 23
    is God's love, 6
    is in all things, 86
    is law that governs all things, 86
    is law which governs all things, 36
    is Spirit of Christ, 7
    is truth, 69
    of Christ, 63
    of God's love infuses joy, 41
    of the body is the eye, 129
    return to original ... we had with the Father, 127
    reveals deeds of darkness, 129
    variations of, 20
Light of Christ, 63
Lord Omnipotent, 85
lot
    casting our lot with Jesus Christ, 138
love, 16, 32, 38, 41-43, 95, 99, 101
    amount of God's ... we feel at judgment not related to worthines, 167
loving feelings, 172

M

man
    also in the beginning with God, 105
    was in the beginning with God, 79, 105
mass, 11, 19
matter, 20, 27, 30, 51
    all spirit is, 27
    eternity of, 25
    intelligence, spirit, ..., elements, law all variations of light, 20
    intelligence, spirit, ..., elements, law have diff. properties, 20
    is also energy, 23
    is element in which all glory dwells, 80
    life in all, 24, 25
    organize, 37
    physical, 27
Melvin Morse, 18
men
    just ... made perfect through Jesus Christ, 182
    receive wages of whom they list to obey, 130
mercy, 7, 16, 30, 32, 38, 93, 95, 98, 99, 101, 127
    claims all which is her own, 100
    has compassion on, 101
mind, 10

minds, 16
Mormonism
    teaches God is finite glorified being with infinite attributes, 31
    view of the other side of life, 46
Mormons, 46
    as non-Christians, 30
Moroni, 157
Moses, 2-4, 35, 36, 45, 111, 143
mourn
    willing to ... with those that, 153
mysteries, 5, 6
mystery of God
    same as mystery of light, energy, matter, 28

N

nature of God
    both infinite and finite, 30
Neal A. Maxwell, 40
near-death experiences, 45
    and beings of light, 46
    and Jesus Christ, 52
    and love, 47, 51, 52
    and mercy, 52
    and omnipresence of God, 50
    and omniscience of God, 50
    and peace, 51, 52
    Andrew Petro, 183
    Carol Zaleski, 182
    Charles Flynn, 184
    Christ is glory and light, 53
    Did you learn to love?, 172
    George Ritchie, 170
    I become the Light, 183
    importance of learning charity for self and others, 170
    Kenneth Ring, 183
    Margot Grey, 183
    matter, 51
    spirit, 51
    support life review after death, 168
    time, 51
    total knowledge, 50
    What knowledge did you gain?, 172
Nephi, 41, 45, 89, 90, 131, 145
nuclear force
    strong, 12
    weak, 12, 16

O

obedience, 97
    I will be obedient, 160

obedient, 80
Oliver Cowdery, 2, 48, 102
omnipotence of God the Father, 36, 38, 87
omnipresence of God the Father, 33, 38, 87
omnipresent, 38
omnipresent energy, 35
omniscience of God the Father, 34, 38
Only Begotten
    By mine ... I created these things, 84
Only Begotten Son, 3, 61, 84, 102
    first great hope of light to Adam and Eve, 136
    full of grace, equity, truth, patience, mercy, 93
opposites, 60, 81
    we live in a world of, 146
opposition in all things, 123
ordinances and covenants
    create a new being through the power of our words, 160
    performing and administering, 161
Orson Pratt, 26, 34, 78, 168

P

Parley P. Pratt, 19, 20, 62, 110
particle, 30, 37, 59, 81, 189
    form, 17, 29, 191, 194
particles
    cannot be diminished or annihilated, 20
patience, 93
patterns
    interference, 192
    photoelectric, 191
Paul, 2, 85
peace, 145, 186
perdition
    darkness of, 110
perfect
    being made ... means receiving our full inheritance as God's, 166
    commanded to be ... like God the Father, 165
    just men made ... through Jesus Christ, 182
    part of being ... is being made ... in one with God and his Son, 186
perfection
    and progression not mutually exclusive concepts, 41
physical death, 127
plan, eternal
    that Jesus Christ be our Savior, 113

power, 11, 32
   in suffering comes from humbly opening heart to accept grace, 148
   of God, 7
priesthood, 7
   holds the keys of the mysteries of God, 159
   is power to direct blessings of God's glory upon us, 158
   is the power; ordinances are physical acts and covenants, 159
progression, 41, 43
   perfection and ... not mutually exclusive concepts, 41

R

radio waves, 20
Raymond Moody, 46
remission of sins
   retaining a ... from day to day, 153
resurrection
   unites energy light of our spirit with material light of body, 181
   unites spirits of light with bodies of light, 181
return
   to original light we had with the Father, 127
reuniting heaven and earth, 177

S

sacrament
   we become part of Christ through, 158
sacrament table
   we eat and drink the fruit of the tree of life, 146
sacrifice, 42
   lifts us toward the likeness of God the Father, 43
   lifts us toward the likeness of our Elder Brother, Jesus Christ, 43
sanctification
   by Holy Ghost, 157
Satan, 3, 40
   angel of God in authority, 114
   darkness of, 3
   first act of agency was a lie, 113
   liar from the beginning, 111
   rebelled against God, 113
   wages of ... is darkness, 132
Savior, 90, 103
   promise of a, 120
Second Comforter, 173
   don't have to wait until the resurrection to receive, 174
   is to have the personage of Jesus Christ to attend you, 174
   last Comforter, 174
   reveals mysteries of Godliness, 175
Second Coming
   of Lord Jesus Christ, 103
   sign of the Son of Man, 103
   time when Christ will reveal all his light, 103
Sidney Ridgon, 175
Sidney Rigdon, 6, 102
sons and daughters
   in similitude of Only Begotten, 5
   we are also ... of God, 5
   we become ... of Jesus Christ, 64
sorrow
   of the atonement, 97
sound waves, 13
space
   all ... is filled with elements, 25
spirit, 10, 16, 20, 30, 51
   /matter, 21
   all ... is matter, 27
   intelligence, ..., matter, elements, law all variations of light, 20
   intelligence, ..., matter, elements, law have diff. properties, 20
   matter, 27
Spirit of Christ, 7, 63
spirit of man
   every ... was innocent in the beginning, 142
Spirit of Truth, 105, 106
spiritual
   bodies, 110
   element, 110
   light, 15
   world, 119
Stephen Hawking, 19
Stephen Robinson, 142
Steven, 2
study of light includes
   celestial kingdoms, 11
   compassion, 11
   death, 11
   energy, 11
   grace, 11
   intelligence, 11
   judgment, 11
   knowledge, 11
   laws, 11

life, 11
love, 11
matter, 11
opposites, 11
priesthood, 11
sorrow, 11
subatomic particles, 20
subatomic parts, 23
    both wave and particle, 23
    interconnected, 24
suffering
    can open us to sympathize with the pains of others, 148

T

temple, 161
    a place where we can bring our righteous acts, 160
temples, 45
time, 39, 40
    came into being when God organized space & matter out of energy, 39
    many "times" equal one "time" with God, 39
    varies according to how fast a planet or solar system travels, 82
    varies according to how much gravity is present, 82
tree
    of knowledge of good and evil, 83, 124, 171
    of life (light), 124
Tree of Life, 41
    body and blood of Jesus Christ, 130
    fruit of, 137
    lest Adam put forth his hand, eat, and live forever, 127
truth, 7, 38, 91, 93, 95
    all ..., including love, is light, 2
    has two faces (wave and particle, energy and matter, ...), 28
    is independent, 106
    is knowledge, 35
    is light, 20
    is Spirit of Jesus Christ, 20
    must cleave to truth, 101
    word of the Lord is, 84

U

Urim and Thummim, 179

V

variations of light
    elements, 20
    intelligence, 20
    law, 20
    matter, 20
    radio waves, 20
    spirit, 20
    subatomic particles, 20
    visual light, 20
    x-rays, 20
veil, 28, 39
Viktor Frankl, 146
Virgin Mary, 89
virtue, 7
visual light, 20

W

wave, 15, 16, 30, 59, 81, 189
    form, 29, 190, 193, 194
wave/particle, 21
    dichotomy, 18
    duality, 18, 24
waves, 13, 17
wholeness
    uniting spirit bodies with physical bodies into celestial light, 184
Word, 84
    in the beginning the ... was, 90
    in the beginning with God, 84
    Jesus Christ was the ... that was made flesh, 97
work, 11

X

x-rays, 13, 20